Praise for Michael Callen's *Surviving AIDS*

"Callen captures the spirit and eccentricities of men and women who, shouldering an extraordinary burden, simply will not break."

—*New York Times*

"Passionate. . . . [These] long-term survivors' stories are poignant, angry and/or funny, and their voices—like Callen's—are winning."

—*People*

"A valuable, hope-giving manual."

—*Publishers Weekly*

"A tightly written and frequently witty study celebrating the views of long-term AIDS survivors who are still enjoying life and have no plans to die in the near future."

—*Kirkus Reviews*

"Passionate and informative . . . Callen's audacious enthusiasm for life, his righteous indignation is infectious."

—*Kansas City Star*

"A wonderful hybrid that's part autobiography, part expose, and part self-help book."

—*L.A. Style*

"An inspiring thread of similarities, choices, and courageous paths shared by the author and the people he interviews."

—*Washington Blade*

"Read [these] interviews for their messages courage, strength, and hope."

—*Lambda Book Review*

D0911661

SURVIVING AIDS

Michael Callen

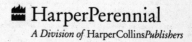 HarperPerennial

A Division of HarperCollins*Publishers*

The Library of Congress has catalogued the hardcover edition as follows:

Callen, Michael, 1955–
    Surviving AIDS / Michael Callen.—1st ed.
        p.   cm.
    Includes bibliographical references.
    ISBN 0-06-016148-5
    1. AIDS (disease)—Patients—United States—Biography.   I. Title.
RC607.A26C33   1990
362.1′969792′0092273—dc20   89-45636
[B]

ISBN 0-06-092125-0 (pbk.)
    92 93 94 95 CC/RRD 10 9 8 7 6 5 4 3 2

With love and gratitude,
I dedicate this book to the
two men in my life
without whose love and support
I might not be here:

Richard Dworkin

Dr. Joseph A. Sonnabend

CONTENTS

THANKS

☒☒☒ Neither the author nor this book would exist if it weren't for my lover, Richard Dworkin, and my doctor and friend, Joseph Sonnabend.

Besides Richard and Joe, the following individuals read various drafts of this book and offered their insightful comments: Patrick Kelly; Celia Farber; David Corkery—an unsung hero of this epidemic; finally, Richard Goldstein of the *Village Voice,* who edited my first article on survival, which became the basis for this book.

The following individuals also helped make this book possible: all those long-term survivors whom I interviewed, especially those whose stories, due to space limitations, didn't make it into the book; all the photographers who let me use their portraits of survivors—especially Jane Rosett; all the cartoonists who graciously gave me permission to reprint their wonderful work; Joy Chiavetta; and all the researchers and physicians interviewed for this book, especially Drs. Ann Hardy and Richard Rothenberg of the Centers for Disease Control.

The following friends and family endured my many bad moods and unreturned phone calls as I chafed against various deadlines: the Flirtations, aka Jon Arterton, Aurelio Font, T. J. Myers, Clifford Townsend, and Rachel Lampert Squires; Carl Valentino; the Board of Directors, the Institutional Review Board, and the staff at the Community Research Initiative (New York); my family, especially Mom and Dad; and my brother-in-"law," Andy Dworkin.

I'd like to thank my agent, Eric Ashworth. At HarperCollins, I'd like to thank my editor, Craig Nelson, his assistant editor, Jennifer Hull, and Matthew Martin, Esq. They made the process of writing this tome comparatively painless.

Finally, feminism—in particular, feminist critiques of the health care system—helped me make some sense of the madness that swirls around me daily. I'd especially like to acknowledge with gratitude the women, particularly the lesbians, who have labored so thanklessly in the struggle to end AIDS.

This book is not a medical manual but rather is intended to present the methods and approaches by which some people are living with and indeed surviving AIDS. Our knowledge about AIDS is uncertain and constantly changing. At this time no one has all the answers, including the author of this book, who is neither a medical doctor nor a scientist. People with AIDS are encouraged to seek the advice and counsel of a variety of qualified medical professionals. The author and the publisher expressly disclaim liability arising from the use or application of any treatments discussed in this book.

INTRODUCTION

"Fighting for Our Lives"

▨▨▨ I was diagnosed with AIDS before the term AIDS even existed. It's been nearly eight years since a doctor told me I had what was then known as GRID—Gay Related Immune Deficiency.

According to the best estimate,[1] of the 1,049 Americans diagnosed with AIDS during 1982, twenty-five are still alive.

I am one of the lucky ones.

From the first description of cases in the *New York Native* in the spring of 1981, there was never any question in my mind that I would get GRID. I retain a clear image of myself on a subway platform at rush hour, frozen in place, reading for the first time about a new, lethal, sexually transmitted disease that was affecting gay men. I remember feeling disoriented by the knowledge that life was going on all around me, oblivious to the fact that my world had just changed utterly and forever.

By late 1981 I was already experiencing mysterious fevers, night sweats, fatigue, rashes, and relentless, debilitating diarrhea. I was losing weight and feeling more and more miserable. Although I didn't get my official AIDS diagnosis until a year later, my doctor and I both knew by the fall of 1981 that I had GRID.

In June 1982, I collapsed from dehydration and was admitted to the hospital with a high fever and violent, bloody diarrhea. When a doctor walked into my hospital room and announced, with the satisfaction of Miss Marple, that it was now official, I was strangely relieved.

"Well, it's GRID all right," she said. "You have cryptosporidiosis. Before GRID, we didn't think cryptosporidiosis infected humans. It's a disease previously found only in livestock."

I tried to take in the fact that I had a disease of *cattle!*

"I'm afraid there is no known treatment. . . ."

I thought I was prepared for this moment, but I felt myself beginning to go numb.

"All we can do is try to keep you hydrated and see what happens. Your body will either handle it or . . . it won't."

She smiled, not too optimistically, patted my leg, and left me alone to confront in earnest the very real possibility of my imminent death.

⊠ Like some rabid animal, AIDS picked me up by the scruff of my neck, shook me senseless, and spat me out forever changed. I am today a totally different person than I was when the decade and the epidemic began. AIDS has been a cosmic kick in the ass—a challenge to *finally* begin living fully.

I was all of twenty-seven when I was diagnosed with AIDS.

At the time, I had been transformed from a silly, immature, lonely Midwesterner into a silly, immature, lonely urban gay man. I had acquaintances—mainly from work—but no real friends. My life consisted of work and sex. Although when asked I told everyone I was a singer, I worked by day as a legal secretary. I only halfheartedly pursued singing. There were too many other distractions—mostly sex.

Because I believe that it was the *way* I was gay—the particular gay life-style that I lived in the seventies—that led to my getting AIDS,[2] I want to chart the path that led to that hospital bed in 1982.

Prior to the gay liberation movement, gay people looked in the mirror of American culture and never—not once—saw our image accurately reflected. It's easy now, when lesbian couples attend high school proms and openly gay people are elected to Congress, to forget what it was like to be homosexual before gay liberation—particularly if you didn't live in a major city on either coast.

For the first seventeen years of my life, I never traveled outside of a sixty-mile radius of the small Indiana town I'd been born in. I was fourteen the first time I ever *heard* the word "homosexual." I was playing canasta with three girls when the oldest narrowed her eyes, pointed at me, and declared with great authority: "If you don't stop acting like a girl, you're gonna turn into a homosexual."

I didn't know what the word meant, but I broke out in a cold sweat. Instinctively, I knew that a homosexual must be *the* most horrible thing anyone could ever be—so horrible that no one had ever spoken of it in my presence.

In the middle of a sermon at the Methodist church my family regularly attended, it dawned on me that "homosexual" was the adult word for "men who burn with lust towards other men."[3] If I "turned into" a homosexual, I was doomed to hell.

I looked up homosexuality in a psychology textbook and found it in the chapter on deviance, alongside murderers, pedophiles, and kleptomaniacs.

I went to Woolworth's, bought a copy of Dr. David Reuben's *Everything You Always Wanted to Know About Sex, But Were Afraid to Ask,*[4] and hid it in the attic. I can still see myself, heart pounding and mouth dry, reading the book and feeling as if my future was being revealed to me. The book said that men who felt like I did were pathetic psychopaths who hung out in public rest rooms writing lurid notes to each other on toilet paper.

I know it seems crazy, but I really believed what I read in *Everything You Always Wanted to Know About Sex.* After all, it was written by an expert, and an M.D. to boot. It was a best-seller. It *had* to be true. Using the only information I had about how to find others like me, I had my first consciously gay sexual experience in a filthy public toilet in Boston shortly after I'd enrolled at Boston University. The only information I had said that all gay men were promiscuous, and so I was.

▓ Had it not been for the gay liberation movement, I would probably have lived out the rest of my life fulfilling every one of Dr. Reuben's inhuman stereotypes about homosexual men.

It wasn't until my junior year of college that I discovered gay liberation. I accidentally stumbled into a meeting of the Boston University gay student group.

It was a revelation. I learned that there were millions of others like me. It was life-changing to discover that the horrible things mainstream society was saying about us—things I had internalized—were not true.

I came out with a vengeance. I did battle with everyone, especially my parents. For a year, I wouldn't speak to my father. I was bitter and abrasive, rigid and impatient.

▓ At first, I had been promiscuous because the only information I had about gay men was that we were all promiscuous *by nature.* But after discovering gay liberation, I proudly and defiantly celebrated the promiscuity that mainstream society so disapproved of.

Although the lesbian and gay political agenda was much broader than sex, I was only interested in the part that dealt with pleasure. One strain of seventies gay liberationist rhetoric proclaimed that sex was inherently liberating; by a curiously naive calculus, it seemed to follow that *more* sex was *more* liberating. In other words, I should consider myself more liberated if I'd had a thousand sex partners than if I'd only had five hundred.

Some of us believed we could change the world through sexual liberation and that we were taking part in a noble experiment. Certain gay theorists argued that there was powerful potential for political change inherent in a brotherhood of lust. Where else, they argued, could a Wall Street stockbroker and a Puerto Rican delivery boy, each divested of the costumes and privileges of rank and class, "come together" as equals? The situation seemed positively *charged* with radical potential.

The opportunities for gay men to have sex with each other multiplied during the seventies at an unprecedented rate, as did peer pressure to partake of these fruits of gay liberation. Never before had so many men had so much sex with so many different partners.

During the seventies, I considered myself a lowly private doing battle on the front lines of the sexual revolution. I joked that I was a fast-food sex junkie. For me, being gay *meant* having lots of sex.

In a lecture I attended on the eve of the age of AIDS, one of my favorite writers, Edmund White, co-author of *The Joy of Gay Sex,* proposed that "gay men should wear their sexually transmitted diseases like red badges of courage in a war against a sex-negative society." I remember nodding my head in vigorous agreement and saying to myself, "Gee! Every time I get the clap I'm striking a blow for the sexual revolution!"

Unfortunately, as a function of a microbiological, not a moral, certainty, this level of sexual activity resulted in concurrent epidemics of syphilis, gonorrhea, hepatitis, amebiasis, venereal warts and, we discovered too late, other pathogens.[5] Unwittingly, and with the best of revolutionary intentions, a small subset of gay men managed to create disease settings equivalent to those of poor third-world nations in one of the richest nations on earth.

▨ This is the road that led to my being diagnosed with AIDS in 1982. The reason I have dwelt on promiscuity is that I believe that I'm still alive because at a crucial point in my illness I was willing to confront some harsh realities about the life I had led. I became convinced that I had overloaded my immune system one too many times with the many sexually transmitted diseases I had as a result of my promiscuity.

My controversial beliefs about the cause of AIDS have been strongly influenced by my doctor, Joe Sonnabend. Following the first reports of GRID in the spring of 1981, Dr. Sonnabend began to formulate a multifactorial theory about what might be causing it.[6] Based on his firsthand knowledge of the life-styles and disease histories of the gay men in his practice who were getting this new disease, he proposed that it was the repeated assaults on the immune system by a *variety of common* sexually transmitted infectious (and other noninfectious) factors that, over time, were resulting in a profound, sustained immune deficiency.[7]

An early Centers for Disease Control (CDC) report[8] indicating that the median number of lifetime sexual partners for the first 100 gay men with AIDS was a staggering 1,120 supported Joe's theory that repeated infection with sexually transmitted diseases might be playing a crucial role in making people sick. Early T-cell testing on thirty of his patients further confirmed Joe's suspicions. Those patients who were monogamous had normal immune function; those who occasionally ran in the fast lane had minor degrees of immune dysfunction; and those of us with a long history of sexually transmitted disease were profoundly immune-deficient.[9]

Joe believed that AIDS in other so-called risk groups was most likely caused by a similar multifactorial process, although the specific infections and other immunosuppressive factors might be different than those for gay men.

Today, of course, most people believe that AIDS is caused by the human immunodeficiency virus (HIV).[10] Proponents of the HIV theory believe that the staggering list of common sexually transmitted diseases that accompanied the fabled promiscuity of the late seventies had nothing to do with *causing* AIDS in gay men. Promiscuity may have helped HIV spread faster, they admit, but it's certainly not the *cause* of AIDS.

▨ It wasn't until I was officially diagnosed with AIDS that I faced squarely just how much sex, and how much disease, I'd had.

With the gentle prodding of a doctor who was filling out my CDC AIDS case report form, I calculated that since becoming sexually active in 1973, I had racked up more than three thousand different sex partners in bathhouses, back rooms, meat racks, and tearooms. As a consequence, I had also had the following sexually transmitted diseases, many more than once: hepatitis A, hepatitis B, hepatitis non-A/non-B; herpes simplex types I and II; venereal warts; amebiasis, including giardia lamblia and entamoeba histolytica; shigella flexneri and salmonella; syphilis; gonorrhea; nonspecific urethritis; chlamydia; cytomegalovirus (CMV), and Epstein-Barr virus (EBV) mononucleosis; and eventually cryptosporidiosis and, therefore, AIDS.

The question in my mind became not so much why I had AIDS, but how I had been able to remain standing on two feet for so long.

Before I discovered Joe's multifactorial theory, much of my postdiagnosis depression came from my belief that I was a ticking time bomb—that some as yet unidentified killer virus inside me was slowly and inexorably destroying my immune system. Because they hadn't even identified any such virus in 1982, I felt helpless. And I knew that even if an AIDS virus was eventually found, there probably wouldn't be a treatment for it within my lifetime, because there weren't many effective treatments for other viral infections. Believing that a killer virus was responsible for my illness made my survival prospects seem grim and sapped my will to put up a fight.

Whether or not Joe's multifactorial theory of AIDS ultimately proves to be correct, discovering a different way of thinking about AIDS at such a crucial turning point in my life provided a framework for me to justify believing that I might survive my disease. It was a life raft that kept me afloat in a sea of doom and gloom.

⊠ But back in 1982, whether one believed that AIDS was being caused by repeated infection with the STDs that plagued gay men or that promiscuity was simply the means by which some killer virus was being spread, something needed to be done—and no one was doing it. Gay leadership seemed paralyzed by the mind-boggling prospect that unforeseen consequences of the sexual freedoms we'd fought so hard for might now be killing us.

To Dr. Sonnabend and to me, what needed to be done was clear: Gay men needed to be warned in no uncertain terms that if they continued to pursue life-styles that abused their immune systems, they might die. Gay men would have to radically alter their sexual behavior. And this impossible task would have to be accomplished virtually overnight. Someone needed to issue the call to arms for a *second* sexual revolution.

⊠ Writing with the moral force of two self-identified "AIDS victims" (the term "people with AIDS" hadn't been invented yet), Richard Berkowitz (another of Joe's patients) and I entered the AIDS political fray in November 1982 with an article published in a New York City gay newspaper entitled "We Know Who We Are: Two Gay Men Declare War on Promiscuity."[11]

Based on Dr. Sonnabend's multifactorial theory, it was a blunt, provocative warning to gay men about the possible consequences of continuing to expose themselves to the diseases that were epidemic among promiscuous gay men. With the frenzy of recently reformed whores singing gospel, we were *testifying* about the urgent need to "avoid the exchange of potentially infectious bodily fluids."

Going public with the suggestion that life-style played any role in the development of AIDS set off a fire storm of protest. Undaunted, I took my income tax refund and published a widely disseminated follow-up, a forty-eight-page booklet entitled *How to Have Sex in an Epidemic: One Approach.*[12] *How to Have Sex* was among the first publications, if not the first,[13] to introduce the concept of safe sex. (The "r" was added to "safe" later, to appease the conservatives who maintained that there was no such thing as risk-free sex—only risk-reduced sex.)

Although "avoiding the exchange of potentially infectious bodily fluids" has now become the accepted standard of AIDS risk reduction, we were harshly criticized—especially by the Gay Men's Health Crisis (GMHC)—when we first proposed it.[14] We believed that the advice GMHC was then giving gay men—to reduce the number of sex partners and to "know" one's partners—was dangerously inadequate. GMHC and other critics retorted that by focusing attention on the incidence of the many sexually transmitted diseases common among promiscuous gay men, we were "shouting guilt from the rooftops."[15] A GMHC board member, who wrote about AIDS for the most widely read national gay publication, referred to our "vigilante impulsivity" and claimed that we were urging gay men to "follow along in self-flagellation."[16]

It was hard enough to be sick and fighting for my own life. To be attacked for trying to save the lives of others was deeply wounding. But we felt we had no choice. The message that gay men had to change the way they were having sex simply had to get out.

▨ Fortunately, even my harshest critics and I agreed that there was an urgent need to attack the homophobia and apathy that characterized the federal government's inadequate response to AIDS. In addition to preaching the gospel of safer sex, I joined the fight against the injustice of the pathetic federal response to AIDS. After years as a law-abiding, tax-paying citizen, I was incensed that my government's virtual nonresponse to AIDS starkly demonstrated that America didn't care whether people like me lived or died.

By the end of the decade, I had testified before every legislative body that would listen, from city council subcommittees to the United States Congress. I was the first publicly identified PWA to meet with representatives of the White House.

What motivated my political activism during this period was a desire to put a human face on AIDS. A handful of other PWAs and I believed that if we could convince the so-called general population that AIDS was happening to real people, not faceless "risk groups," we could awaken Americans to the need for an all-out war against this disease.

Over the years, I've done a mind-boggling amount of PWA public relations. I debated Rock Hudson's ex-lover on Phil Donahue, was featured in early profiles in *New York* magazine and *Life,* and did hundreds of interviews for radio, TV, and print media.

Those of us crazy enough to publicly identify ourselves as having the most stigmatized disease of the century agreed that it felt strange to be treated like "celebrities" for having AIDS. Only in America, I thought, would it be necessary to make a career out of being sick in order to compel a more humane and appropriate government response.

In San Francisco, Los Angeles, and other cities, other PWAs such as Bobbi Campbell and Dan Turner were fighting similar battles. The PWA self-empowerment movement was born when a dozen of us met for the first time at a historic AIDS conference held in Denver in 1983. Once we were in the same room, we discovered that we had similar complaints: No one was listening to us or taking us seriously.

We drafted the founding manifesto of the people with AIDS self-empowerment movement, which became known as "The Denver Principles." Bobbi Campbell and I wrote the first draft on the back of some old handbills.

Our opening statement made clear our resolve to fight back against the powerful forces that were trying to dehumanize us:

> We condemn attempts to label us as "victims," a term which implies defeat, and we are only occasionally "patients," a term which implies passivity, helplessness and dependence upon the care of others. We are "People With AIDS."[17]

Prior to Denver, those of us *with* AIDS had had no voice in the AIDS organizations that had been set up to help us. The concept of PWA self-empowerment hammered out in Denver by a group of feisty PWAs was radical in its simplicity: People with AIDS should have a say in any decision-making process that will affect our lives. It was the AIDS equivalent of the principle of "No taxation without representation."

▨ Returning from Denver, electrified by the righteousness of the cause of PWA self-empowerment, a group of us founded the first political organization of people with AIDS in New York City. We immediately fell into bitter warfare with the Gay Men's Health Crisis. GMHC was not about to permit a bunch of upstart, radical "clients" to tell them how to run their operation. (Despite the fact that the Denver principles demanded that PWAs "be involved at every level of decision-making and specifically serve on the boards of directors of provider organizations," GMHC did not add a publicly identified person with AIDS to its board of directors until 1987.)

Ultimately, GMHC succeeded in destroying the first organized incarnation of PWA self-empowerment in New York through a two-pronged strategy of alternately ignoring and ridiculing us. But out of the ashes of the first PWA group, we formed the PWA Coalition. Today, the Coalition continues to provide important services to people with AIDS and has an annual budget approaching $1 million.

I became the founding editor of the PWA Coalition *Newsline*, a newsletter written almost entirely by people with AIDS. What started out as a ragged newsletter has turned into a slick, lively forum for the diverse opinions of people with AIDS. Fifteen thousand copies are printed and mailed out each month to PWAs around the world.

Selecting from the best writing published in the *Newsline*, I edited two volumes of "helpful hints" for the newly diagnosed, published by the PWA Coalition under the title *Surviving and Thriving with AIDS*.

▨ Throughout these early years, my extraordinary relationship with Dr. Sonnabend extended far beyond his medical management of my illness. We co-authored a number of provocative, controversial articles. Together, we have been involved in the founding of several major AIDS organizations, including the AIDS Medical Foundation, which later became the American Foundation for AIDS Research (AmFAR).

Together with Tom Hannan, we founded the People with AIDS Health Group. The Health Group operates like a co-op to import, essentially at cost, drugs that are unavailable in the United States.

The most recent project Joe and I (and others) embarked on was the founding of the Community Research Initiative. CRI conducts rigorous scientific research on promising AIDS therapies in a community-based setting faster and more cheaply than traditional systems do. Also, CRI utilizes study designs that are sensitive to the needs of PWAs, because PWAs and the physicians who care for us are involved at every level of the decision-making process: on the Institutional Review Board, the Board of Directors, the Scientific Advisory Committee, and on staff.

When we first proposed the idea of community-based research, everyone said that it was too ambitious, it couldn't be done. We were told that medical centers, with their monopoly on drug research, would never allow such upstart competition. Once again, skeptics have been proven wrong.

There is now a network of more than forty community-based research centers in the United States, with similar organizations being set up in other countries.[18] If the community-based research movement accomplishes nothing else, its successful conduct of the research that led to FDA approval of aerosolized pentamidine, for the prevention of the pneumonia that is the number-one killer of people with AIDS, more than justifies the backbreaking effort it took to launch it.

◼ While I would never have wished for AIDS, the plain truth is that I'm happier now than I've ever been. Having AIDS has been like going through ten years of therapy—every week.

AIDS has taught me the preciousness of life and the healing power of love. I've been more productive than at any time prior. I've traveled the world and met hundreds of wonderful people that I'm sure I would not have met any other way. I've tried to see AIDS as a challenge to begin living, instead of a sign to begin dying.

AIDS forced me to take responsibility for my own life—for the choices I had made and the choices I could still make. For better or worse, AIDS has made me the man I am today.

◼ I have tried to help shape how America thinks about—and responds to—AIDS. I have done what I've done out of a sincere belief that suffering could be reduced and lives could be saved.

The common thread that has run through my AIDS activism has been a passionate belief that hopelessness kills. That is why challenging the myth that everyone dies from AIDS has become an obsession.

The slogan of the PWA self-empowerment movement is "Fighting for

Our Lives." For the last eight years, that is precisely what I've been doing. I have fought with the viciousness of a cornered animal that knows if it loses a battle, it loses its life. Since I was diagnosed with AIDS, I've made it my mission to fight back against the hopelessness and gloom that pervade AIDS and that sap the will to live.

If I believed everything I was told—if I had believed that tiresome boilerplate lie that AIDS is 100 percent fatal—I'd probably be dead by now. If I didn't arm myself with information—facts, statistics, and diverse views—I would be unable to defend myself against the madness and gibberish that daily assault those of us who have AIDS.

This book is the result of three and a half years of trying to understand the mystery of long-term survival—my own as well as that of others. It presents the collected wisdom of dozens of survivors.

We survivors must bear witness to the horrors we have endured. But even as we grieve, even as we honor the memory of those who have fallen, we must at the same time fix our hearts and minds on a clear image of the day when AIDS is no more.

Make no mistake about it; that day will come.

NOTES

1. According to James Buehler of the Centers for Disease Control, statistics current as of February 1, 1990, indicate that between January and June of 1982, 385 cases were reported nationally, of which 90.6 percent are dead. That means thirty-six people are still listed as alive. Between July and December of 1982, 664 cases were reported, 89.3 percent of whom are known to have died. That means seventy-one of those diagnosed in the second half of 1982 are still listed as being alive.

Therefore, the CDC lists 107 people as potentially still alive from the 1049 who were diagnosed with AIDS in 1982. I have arrived at my best guess of twenty-six of us *actually* alive by reducing the 107 figure by 75 percent, roughly the percentage of PWAs still listed as alive but who, through intensive follow-up, were found to have actually died in a study on long-term survival performed by Dr. Ann Hardy. This study is discussed in the chapter that follows, Just the Facts, Ma'am.

2. One of the things I hate most about living as a gay man in a deeply homophobic society is what I call the myth of the homogenous homosexual—the absurd notion that all gay men are alike. Just as is true of heterosexuals, gay men lead very different life-styles. As I discuss elsewhere, I suspect that only a small minority of gay men ever partook of the fast-lane life-style that I led. A friend of mine who died of AIDS early in the epidemic put it this way: "Being gay doesn't make you sick; it's being a *pig* about it."

3. Romans I:26–27, from the Bible (authorship attributed to God, circa the thirteenth century B.C.). See also Leviticus 18:22–23 and 20:13, King James version.

4. Reuben, David, M.D. *Everything You Always Wanted to Know About Sex, But Were Afraid to Ask.* New York: David McKay Publishers, 1969. See his deeply homophobic, egregiously misinformed chapter on homosexuality.

5. Although statistics documenting an alarming rise in epidemics of sexually transmitted diseases among gay men were readily available prior to AIDS (see *Sexually Transmitted Diseases in Homosexual Men: Diagnosis, Treatment, and Research,* David G. Ostrow, Terry Alan Sandholzer, and Yehudi Felman, eds. New York: Plenum Medical Book Company, 1983), no one took heed of the warning signs that were all around us. No one asked what the cumulative consequences might be of continually wallowing in what was, to put it bluntly, an increasingly polluted microbiological sewer. Rumors that the Health Department had been able to culture cholera and other exotic microbes from the greasy stair rails of the Mineshaft (a notorious Manhattan sex club) were dismissed as apocryphal.

We took each new disease in stride. I can even recall that the "invention" of a disease dubbed as "gay bowel syndrome" was, in some quarters, almost a matter of pride; now we even had our own *diseases,* just like we had our own plumbers and tax advisers. A whole new breed of physicians, affectionately known as "clap doctors," grew rich treating our STDs. Many of these physicians could themselves be observed in the bathhouses and back rooms leading the same fast-lane life-style as their patients. Even if they had warned us, who would have listened?

We thought of our bodies as machines to be perfected at the gym; when they'd break down, our doctors would give us some medicine and we'd go back into the breach as good as new. It seems astounding that we failed to notice that the conditions which facilitated the transmission of bacteria and parasites—infectious agents for which there usually were effective treatments—were the same conditions which also facilitated the transmission of viruses—pathogens for which there were few, if any, proven therapies.

We didn't think about what the long-term consequences of repeated reinfection with common viruses might be or what would happen if a new germ entered this environment. Nor did we consider the cumulative effects on our bodies of all the drugs and alcohol we were ingesting. It's heartbreaking to realize that the simple introduction of condoms into the sexual culture of the seventies would have prevented the many epidemics of STDs, including, I believe, AIDS.

6. See Sonnabend, J.A., Witkin, S.S., et al., "Acquired immunodeficiency syndrome: Opportunistic infections and malignancies in male homosexuals," *JAMA (Journal of the American Medical Association),* 249 (1983): 2370. For the latest, updated version of Dr. Sonnabend's multifactorial explanation for AIDS, see Sonnabend, J. A., "AIDS: An Explanation for Its Occurrence in Homosexual Men," in *AIDS and Opportunistic Infections of Homosexual Men,* P. Ma and D. Armstrong, eds. (Stoneham, MA: Butterworth Publishers, 1989).

7. Those interested in understanding Dr. Sonnabend's multifactorial conceptualization of AIDS should definitely read it in the original. (For reference, see preceding note.) However, for those who would like a general overview, Dr. Sonnabend believes that the key factor for the development of AIDS among gay men is repeated infection with cytomegalovirus (CMV), a herpes virus that causes a monolike condition. CMV reached epidemic proportions among sexually active gay men during the late seventies. A single CMV infection is violently immunosuppressive, and evidence suggests one

can be multiply, and repeatedly, infected. CMV infection sets off a cascade of other events, probably including reactivation of Epstein-Barr virus (EBV) and other latent infections. Other immunosuppressive cofactors include untreated, or undertreated, syphilis and other sexually transmitted infections.

Noninfectious cofactors further burdening the immune system of a fast-lane gay man of the seventies included recreational drugs and semen itself (when introduced rectally).

Most people have an unsophisticated view of how people get sick. Many people think that for every disease, there is one specific cause and that getting sick is a simple matter of being infected with the causative agent. That is why so many people equate being infected with HIV—the so-called "AIDS virus"—with actually having AIDS. Such a simplistic view ignores the important distinctions between exposure, infection, and symptomatic disease. Obviously, many people exposed to a germ don't get infected, and many of those infected never go on to get sick. If you put ten people in the same room with someone who has a cold, four people might get the cold and six people won't. The reasons why are multifactorial.

Many people implicitly understand that certain diseases, such as heart disease, are inherently multifactorial. For instance, most people seem to grasp that too much cholesterol can be bad for you. Even so, people who survive a heart attack never ask whether "the cause" of their heart attack was the pat of butter they had on that morning's toast or whether it was caused by the butter they ate ten years ago. With heart disease, people understand that genetics, diet, exercise, and other factors conspire to determine whether or not one will suffer a stroke. But for some reason, most people abandon any notion that getting sick is a multifactorial process once an infectious agent is involved.

For the purpose of the discussion in this chapter, the most important difference between Joe's multifactorial view of the etiology of AIDS and the view that currently prevails is that he does not believe a single event—infection with HIV or any other infectious agent—can account for a disease as complex as AIDS, in which so many immunological systems go haywire.

8. The CDC did not publish its detailed profile of the first cases of AIDS among gay men until 1984. The 1,120 figure, however, was widely known as early as the fall of 1981. A representative of the National Cancer Institute mentioned this figure in an early AIDS lecture. Much to the chagrin of gay leaders at the time, we publicized this figure in our first AIDS missive, "We Know Who We Are: Two Gay Men Declare War on Promiscuity."

9. Wallace, J., Coral, F., Sonnabend, J.A., et al., "T-Cell ratios in homosexuals," *Lancet* 1 (1982): 908.

10. In the early years of the AIDS epidemic—especially prior to 1984, when HIV was declared to be the sole cause of AIDS—the multifactorial theory was considered quite plausible by many of those now convinced that HIV is the cause of AIDS. When HIV was first proposed by French researchers as the cause of AIDS, researchers ignored it. Later, when the U.S. government announced with great fanfare that HIV (then known as HTLV-III) was "the probable cause of AIDS," there was open skepticism on the part of many AIDS researchers and journalists. One important challenge to the assertion that HIV could explain AIDS that has never been answered

is this: Instead of being the cause of AIDS, why isn't it just as likely that HIV is merely another opportunistic infection that has been reactivated from a latent state after whatever is *truly* causing AIDS has led to profound immune deficiency? AIDS is a disease characterized by the frequent reactivation of all latent infections, and since HIV has a latency mechanism, it is important to rule out the possibility that HIV antibody positivity is the *effect*, rather than the cause, of immune deficiency.

In order to stay in the AIDS debate at all, I've had to learn what I call the language of HIV. (I like to think I speak it without much of an accent.) But to this day, I still believe that repeated infection by common sexually transmitted diseases that had reached epidemic levels is a more plausible explanation for the epidemic of AIDS among gay men. Of course, most people still think that my views are outrageous.

There is, of course, a lot of *circumstantial* evidence implicating HIV in the etiology of AIDS. But it is by no means conclusive. As we enter the second decade of AIDS, we still can't say with any reasonable certainty precisely *how* a virus as biochemically inactive as HIV can account for the profound immunodeficiency we now call AIDS. It has become clear that HIV doesn't infect nearly enough T-helper cells to account for their massive destruction in AIDS, and now that the simplistic Pac-man model of HIV T-cell killing has been abandoned, a frantic search is on to find indirect mechanisms of cell killing. It is of course appropriate to continue researching HIV, but not to the exclusion of other, equally promising, theories.

For a fascinating examination of the dire cost of having prematurely closed the debate on the cause of AIDS, see Sonnabend, Joseph, M.D., "Fact and Speculation About the Cause of AIDS," *AIDS Forum*, vol. 2, no. 1 (May 1989): 3–12.

11. Callen, Michael, and Berkowitz, Richard (with Richard Dworkin and Dr. Joseph Sonnabend), "We Know Who We Are: Two Gay Men Declare War on Promiscuity," *New York Native*, November 8–21, 1982.

12. Callen, Michael, and Berkowitz, Richard. *How to Have Sex in an Epidemic: One Approach*, first published in May 1983. Edited by Richard Dworkin with a foreword by Dr. Joseph Sonnabend. This booklet is now out of print. However, significant portions have been reprinted in *Surviving and Thriving with AIDS: Collected Wisdom*, vol. 2. Michael Callen, ed. (New York: PWA Coalition, Inc., 1988), 164–167.

13. San Francisco's Sisters of Perpetual Indulgence had published their famous, ground-breaking "Can We Talk . . ." brochure, which encouraged condom use, at about the same time that we had completed writing *How to Have Sex in an Epidemic: One Approach*.

14. Ironically, the same people who were accusing us of being "sex-negative" on the basis of "We Know Who We Are" saw no inconsistency in also criticizing *How to Have Sex in an Epidemic: One Approach* because they felt that safer sex would encourage promiscuity. We took no stand on the emotional or ethical value of promiscuity. We merely wanted those who chose to continue to be promiscuous in the face of the epidemic to do so *safely*. But since this conflicted with GMHC's advice at the time, we were criticized harshly.

Just for the record, I think promiscuity has its place. I sometimes long nostalgically for what was good about the gay sexual revolution of the seventies—the playfulness and adventure. The point is, whatever sex one chooses to engage in these days, it should be safer sex and, I believe, it should proceed from a loving instinct to communicate with another human being, rather than being about merely scratching a physical itch, with no regard for the humanity of the individual you're scratching the itch with.

Although I have criticized a certain type of promiscuity—the acquisitive, competitive, generally drug-enhanced kind that I practiced in my youth—I believe that promiscuity can be a good thing for some people. I am tremendously intrigued by a new movement that has recently sprung up in the gay community. The essence of this movement is that gay men should use sex to honor themselves and their partners. Instead of recreational drugs, it utilizes full-body massage and rebirthing techniques to enhance and extend sexual pleasure. It celebrates the diversity of the human body and is much less "looks-ist" (to use the awkward feminist phrase) than we were in the seventies.

15. Seitzman, Peter A., M.D., "Guilt and AIDS," *New York Native*, Issue 54, January 3–16, 1983.

16. Fain, Nathan, "Coping with a Crisis: AIDS and the Issues It Raises," *The Advocate*, Issue 361, February 17, 1982.

17. "The Denver Principles, Statement from the Advisory Committee of People with AIDS," reprinted in *Surviving and Thriving with AIDS: Collected Wisdom*, vol. 2. Michael Callen, ed. (New York: PWA Coalition, Inc., 1988), 294–295.

18. For a complete listing of the established and emerging community-based research initiatives in the U.S., contact Paul Corser at the American Foundation for AIDS Research, (212) 719-0033.

1

AIDS: The Present Situation

[A]bout half . . . [of] the number of persons known to have AIDS in the United States . . . have died of the disease. Since there is no cure, the others are expected to also eventually die from their disease.

—Dr. C. Everett Koop, "Surgeon General's Report on Acquired Immune Deficiency Syndrome," U.S. Department of Health and Human Services, undated brochure mailed to every U.S. household

"EXPECTED TO . . . DIE"

▨▨▨ "Max just asked if you were dead yet."

Max is the precocious six-year-old son of the piano player in my lover's jazz band. Max hadn't seen me in several months and so it must have seemed a logical question.

My lover laughed nervously, not knowing what to make of the expression on my face when he told me. I was momentarily paralyzed by the insight that here in America, the one essential fact about AIDS—a notion so simple as to be accessible to a six-year-old—is that everyone who gets it dies. Or in the words of the surgeon general, everyone with AIDS is *"expected . . . to die."*

I did a quick reality check: I have AIDS, but as far as I could tell, I was not dead.

Later that week, I read an article that said that AIDS is invariably fatal—that there are no known survivors. As I sat holding the newspaper in my hands, it dawned on me that I was alive five years after my AIDS diagnosis—several years after I was supposed to be dead. I realized that I could name a half-dozen other friends, many of whom were diagnosed before me, who were surviving and thriving with AIDS.

I got furious! How did the myth get started that everyone who gets AIDS dies, and what were the consequences of this lie? How many other long-term survivors were out there? Why have we survived?

I resolved then to write about the best-kept secret of the epidemic: Not everyone dies from AIDS.

▨ The first thing I did was dig out from the wastebasket the monthly New York City AIDS surveillance data. What I discovered pleasantly shocked me. I *wasn't* crazy! According to the government's own statistics, there *were* long-term survivors.

In the September 1987 issue of the People with AIDS (PWA) *Newsline*, I reported that:

> According to New York City Health Department statistics, as of June 24, 1987, nearly 20 percent of People with AIDS are alive more than three years after diagnosis. Here's the statistical breakdown:
>
> > Of the 17 people diagnosed before 1979, 3 are still alive.
> > Of the 23 people diagnosed before January 1, 1980, 3 are still alive.
> > Of the 48 people diagnosed before January 1, 1981, 5 are still alive.
> > Of the 191 people diagnosed before July 1, 1982, 15 are still alive.
> > Of the 651 people diagnosed before January 1, 1983, 66 of us (I was diagnosed in the summer of '82) are still alive.
> > Of the 1,645 people diagnosed before January 1, 1984, 195 are still alive.
> > Of the 3,380 people diagnosed before January 1, 1985, 672 are still alive.

I knew there was a good chance that problems with record-keeping had exaggerated the survival rates. But, I thought, even if you cut the figures in half, it's still clear that there are others out there who are surviving AIDS.

I wanted to know more.

I wanted to speak with statisticians at the Centers for Disease Control (CDC). Were the New York City statistics accurate? Did more than one out of every ten people diagnosed with AIDS survive three or more years? And if so, what was the source of the myth that there are no survivors of AIDS? Was it the government? Was it the press?

I decided to interview AIDS researchers. Was there something in our blood that differentiated us from those who have died from AIDS? Did they have any explanations to offer?

I also wanted to interview community physicians to see if they had any sense of why some of their patients were surviving while others succumbed quickly.

Finally, I knew that I had to find other long-term survivors and interview them in depth. I was certain that they would provide me with the best sense of why some of us have survived. I placed ads in the PWA *Newsline* seeking other long-term survivors. I sought out survivors whenever I traveled to other cities.

As long-term survivors began to crawl out of the woodwork, I realized that before I interviewed them, I'd have to come up with a list of questions. In order to do that, I would have to do some soul-searching: Why did I think *I* was still alive?

My journey in search of answers to the puzzling mystery of long-term AIDS survival had begun.

JUST THE FACTS, MA'AM

What the Statistics Say

▨▨▨ If the Reagan eighties taught us one thing, it was that a lie endlessly repeated often takes on the force of truth. The lie that AIDS is "invariably fatal" has become part of the mythology that surrounds AIDS. At times, holding a newspaper in my hand or hearing a newscaster blithely deny that I and others like me have survived, I have had to pinch myself to make sure I'm still alive.

Of course, I had obviously survived long past the dire predictions; and I knew others who had survived as long, and longer, than me. But I realized that battling against the ingrained fatalism that clings so tenaciously to AIDS would require an official acknowledgment of the phenomenon of long-term survival by the Centers for Disease Control, the federal agency that polices AIDS. I needed CDC statistics to confirm (and in a sense, affirm) that many of us were surviving AIDS for many years. So I began searching through government statistics for some evidence I might use to appeal the death sentence under which we were all living.

As I began to consider the phenomenon of long-term survival, I realized that I would first have to define what I meant by "long-term." Without knowing much about statistics, I decided to define "long-term" as anyone who had survived twice the current median[1] survival time. In 1987, the median survival time for a gay man with KS was about eighteen months, so I chose thirty-six months (three years) as my arbitrary qualifying point.

Interestingly, when I phoned the CDC, I discovered that they were using the same three-years-or-more definition for long-term survival. According to Dr. Ann Hardy, coordinator of the CDC's national study on long-term AIDS survival,

The choice of three years to qualify as a long-term survivor was somewhat arbitrary. It basically was a doubled median survival, which was around 18

22

months. If we were going to try to characterize long-term survivors, we wanted to be sure we were getting the group that were *really* long-term survivors.

It never occurred to me that some people with AIDS would find this definition of long-term survival offensive. But in response to an ad I placed in the PWA Coalition *Newsline* seeking those "long-term survivors who had survived full-blown AIDS for three years or more," I got a number of testy responses from those who fell short of their three-year anniversary. Dr. Hardy has had similar experiences:

> I still get calls from people with AIDS who say, "I was diagnosed in '84 and you're saying I'm not a survivor. . . ." And I say, "Yes, yes, you *are* a survivor; but I'm sorry; we had to have cutoff dates. That doesn't mean it's not remarkable for someone to have survived 2½ years!"

I am sympathetic to both viewpoints. Yes, it *is* an accomplishment to survive—even for one day—the hostility and physical suffering caused by AIDS. But since many PWAs share my dream of living long enough to see a cure for AIDS, it is legitimate to examine survival trends to see how reasonable it is to hope to survive long enough to benefit from a cure. In the end, I am comfortable with arbitrarily defining "long-term survivor" as anyone who has survived full-blown AIDS for three or more years, and that is the definition I use throughout this book.

After rooting around in the confusing statistics collected by various federal, state, and city agencies, it quickly became clear that indeed there were other long-term survivors. After examining the statistics, my darkest fear—that the half-dozen long-term survivors I happened to know would turn out to be the only survivors there were—was forever defused. The evidence is irrefutable: Hundreds of people have survived AIDS for three or more years. Not everyone dies of AIDS.

▨ But determining precisely how many long-term survivors there are and how much survival probabilities have increased was a much harder task.

There have been three major studies on the subject: one in New York City, led by Dr. Richard Rothenberg; the national CDC study led by Dr. Hardy; and one in San Francisco, led by Dr. George Lemp. Each study was slightly different in methodology, time period examined, and assumptions. Not surprisingly, each study produced divergent estimates of survival probability.

The first major study[2] on long-term survival to be published appeared in the prestigious *New England Journal of Medicine*[3] in November 1987—

nearly two years after it had been initiated. The study occasioned a brief flurry of media attention. Working with the New York City Health Department, CDC researcher Dr. Rothenberg's group discovered that 886 (15.2 percent) of the 5,833 people reported to the New York City AIDS registry through December 31, 1985, were still listed as alive.

The possibility that, prior to AZT and the widespread practice of pneumocystis prevention, 15.2 percent of us had survived five or more years was startling. Researchers and public health officials scratched their heads and confessed, in the words of New York City Commissioner of Health Dr. Stephen Joseph, that this 15 percent figure was "greater than [one] would have intuitively expected it to be."[4]

To their credit, Dr. Rothenberg and his coauthors acknowledged that many of those still listed as being alive might prove to actually be dead. They therefore cautioned that their 15.2-percent five-year survival rate "should be viewed as an upper limit."[5] Subsequent aggressive "vital status" follow-up proved their suspicions correct: A *majority* of those listed in the registry as alive had died.

Meanwhile, back at the CDC, it seems that the left hand did not entirely know what the right hand was doing. In November 1987, as Dr. Rothenberg was releasing his New York City survival results, his CDC colleague in Atlanta, Dr. Ann Hardy, was about midway through her own study of national trends in long-term survival. Although they were aware of each other's work—indeed, the majority of cases analyzed by Dr. Hardy were reported from New York and San Francisco—their failure to agree upon methodologies and time periods makes it difficult to usefully compare their findings.

According to Dr. Hardy, in December of 1986, the idea of assessing national AIDS survival trends, and possibly characterizing long-term survivors, had been enthusiastically proposed by epidemiologists at the CDC. Like Dr. Rothenberg, she began her study by generating a list of the 4,073 cases diagnosed from the beginning of the epidemic (including cases diagnosed retrospectively prior to 1981, when AIDS was first described) through December 31, 1983.

She then searched for everyone who had "not been reported as dead"— or, as she put it, persons with AIDS who were "potentially still alive." To the surprise of many, the computer spit out 821 names.

No one at CDC expected that all 821 would turn out, after aggressive follow-up, to be "actually" alive. The national AIDS surveillance system had been set up hastily and was dependent on individual health departments in all fifty states for accurate case reporting. It was widely suspected and eventually proven that local health department follow-up on subsequent opportunistic complications, including death, was poor.

Another roadblock slowed the completion of this important study. Because of concerns about confidentiality, the CDC to this day does not possess personal identifying information on people with AIDS. Only the local health departments have it. Dr. Hardy therefore had to rely on underfunded, overworked AIDS epidemiologists in each state to conduct the aggressive "vital status" follow-up on the 821 potential survivors.

Despite the formidable logistical difficulties facing Dr. Hardy, she managed to get at least some follow-up information on 780 out of the 821. She was even able to coordinate a smaller, intensive study on a forty-eight-person subset of those found to be alive—a labor-intensive study that required local health department personnel to track down the survivors, explain the study, get informed consent, draw blood, and ascertain disease histories.

In sharp contrast to Dr. Rothenberg's conclusions, Dr. Hardy's results (which as of this writing have not been published) were deeply depressing. Of the 780 potential survivors on whom information was gathered, 474 (61 percent) turned out to be dead. Only 119 people were known to be definitely alive three or more years after diagnosis.

The remaining 187 out of the 780 (approximately 24 percent)[6] were categorized as "lost to follow-up," which meant that the physician or institution that had originally reported the case was unable to confirm or deny whether the person was actually alive.

The best Dr. Hardy could do was to present a survival *range* of 2.8 percent to 7.5 percent.[7]

During the month it took me to track down data from the third major study, I was at a loss to account for the huge difference between Dr. Hardy's discouraging low of 2.8 percent and Dr. Rothenberg's admittedly problematic high of 15.2 percent. When I spoke to Dr. Rothenberg, he said that he thought the true three-year survival rate would be somewhere in the middle—"about 9 percent."

As it turns out, there are two major problems with Dr. Hardy's analysis—both of which she readily acknowledges. First is that the large number lost to follow-up reduces the confidence one can have in the accuracy of the conclusions.

The second problem is that the unavoidable delays in completing follow-up, combined with the method of data analysis chosen, have resulted in a "bias toward *underestimating* true three-year-or-more survival rates."

None of these logistical and statistical methodology problems apply to the third study of survival trends, led by Dr. George Lemp of San Francisco. Dr. Hardy and Dr. Rothenberg both agreed that the best median survival estimates come from San Francisco data analyzed by Dr. Lemp and his colleagues. His group has determined that 9.7 percent of those diagnosed in San Francisco between 1980 and 1985 survived three or more years.[8] The main reason for having greater confidence in Dr. Lemp's estimate that one out of every ten persons with AIDS survived three or more years is that the city of San Francisco has the most efficient and rigorous follow-up. Only 7 percent of the San Francisco cases have been lost to follow-up.

And so, after a long, convoluted journey through a jungle of conflicting statistics, I have confirmed that one in ten of those of us diagnosed in the early days have earned the title of long-term survivor. Though lower than Dr. Rothenberg's 15.2 percent, I'm sure that even this 9.7 percent three-year survival rate must seem to some to be "greater than [one] would have intuitively expected it to be."[9]

If my suspicion proves correct that believing in the *possibility* of surviving AIDS is the necessary precondition of actually surviving AIDS, it is heartbreaking to imagine how different survival rates might be if only the fact that one out of ten had survived beyond expectations had been permitted to become part of the public conception of AIDS.

⊠ Having confirmed that 10 percent have survived AIDS for three years or more, it is useful to examine the survival data more closely to see if any other misconceptions about AIDS can be refuted. In fact, the San Francisco data and the findings of Dr. Hardy's "intensive" study of 48 survivors contradict a number of uncritically held misconceptions about AIDS. Among the data:

There are long-term survivors of PCP.

Out of Dr. Hardy's 48-person study 4[10] had had PCP only and 2 more had had both PCP and KS. So 6 people out of 48 have survived three or more years post-PCP. Since the 71 out of 119 survivors *not* intensively studied by the CDC were matched in all demographic and clinical respects to the 48 who were studied, by inference, approximately 15 people diagnosed with PCP between 1979 and 1983 have survived three or more years. Obviously, one's chances of becoming a long-term survivor after PCP are less than if one's only opportunistic infection is KS;[11] but it's still important to acknowledge that it *is* possible to be a long-term survivor of AIDS even if you've had PCP. (Profiles of two-long term survivors of PCP appear on pages 158 and 163.)

Some people have survived more than a decade with AIDS and are still going strong.

Several people diagnosed with KS in 1978 are still surviving and thriving eleven years later. They have proven that it is possible to live more than a decade with AIDS. If they can do it, why not others?

It is possible to survive AIDS without AZT or other similarly toxic treatments.

The survival of a small number of individuals for more than five years prior to the widespread availability of AZT proves that it is theoretically possible to do so. While we must of course continue to press for treatments, it is important to remember that many people have survived AIDS for years who were diagnosed prior to the introduction of AZT in 1986 and the widespread practice of PCP prophylaxis. Thus, when some people with AIDS pursue holistic approaches to healing or refuse to take experimental medications, we can no longer state categorically that their survival is impossible without Western medicine. While I strongly encourage PCP prophylaxis for those at risk, and further counsel the serious consideration of antiviral and immunomodulating drugs of manageable toxicity, it is interesting to note that the overwhelming majority of long-term survivors I interviewed have refused to take AZT. Many had gambled once with an experimental medication: some decided not to tempt fate a second time, and others expressed the view that "if it ain't broke, don't fix it."[12]

It may be possible to cure oneself of AIDS.

Data from Dr. Hardy's study challenges the assertion that "there has not been a single known case of recovery." According to Dr. Hardy, a few of the long-term survivors "had immunologic studies in the normal range." In the medical literature, there have been sporadic reports of people who have reverted from HIV antibody positive to antibody negative. If, as Dr. Hardy's data suggest, there are people who were infected with HIV and who have had Kaposi's sarcoma, but who, five or more years later, have immune functions in the normal range, can we not say that such individuals have recovered from AIDS? Again, even if this phenomenon is extremely rare, the existence of one case would prove that it is *possible* and would suggest that studying such persons might yield important clues to surviving AIDS. According to

Dr. Rothenberg, "There are ample models in other diseases where a subset of people completely clear infections, leaving no trace of having ever been infected. With most diseases, there will be a subgroup who 'cure' themselves. They will divest themselves of both antigen and antibody."

Some long-term survivors are people of color.

Approximately twelve blacks, five Latinos, and three people whose race was only identified as "other" were included among Dr. Hardy's 119 long-term survivors. The common perception in New York City that people of color die dramatically sooner than white gay men with AIDS may be the result of the confusion caused by the disproportionate number of IV drug users who are people of color. It would appear from Dr. Hardy's data that the majority of these long-term surviving people of color are gay and bisexual, though several share the additional risk factor of IV drug use. It seems that people of color whose sole risk factor is gay/bisexual activity have similar survival rates as do white gay/bisexual men. This surmise is supported by the fact that in San Francisco, a city with very few IV-drug-use-related cases of AIDS, black, Latino, and Asian/Pacific Islanders have essentially identical median survival rates as whites. Thus, it appears that race by itself is not a major determinant of survival probabilities. (Profiles of two black and one Latino gay long-term survivors appear on pages 105, 133, and 152.)

There are IV drug users who have survived three or more years with full-blown AIDS.

Approximately twenty of the 119 long-term survivors in Dr. Hardy's study had identified IV drug use as a risk factor. Clearly gay men without a history of IV drug use have better survival prospects then those with; but it is important to acknowledge that there *are* long-term survivors who contracted AIDS through IV drug use. As mentioned, in San Francisco, people with AIDS who identify IV drug use as their sole risk factor have a one-year median survival rate essentially equivalent to that of gay men. The finding that IV drug users (IVDUs) in San Francisco are surviving as long as gay men is discordant with New York data. A number of factors might account for this difference, and investigation of the factors that affect the survival of IVDUs with AIDS is urgently needed. The only woman who met Dr. Hardy's three-year-or-longer definition of long-term survival was both black and an IV drug user. But according to Dr. Hardy, she was kept alive through extraordinary measures and spent her last year in a hospital with a very poor quality of life. She died within days of reaching the third anniversary of her diagnosis. Dr. Rothenberg's study found that "black women who acquired the disease through intravenous drug abuse . . . had a particularly poor prognosis . . . [31 percent alive at one year and 5 percent at two years]."[13] Understanding why AIDS appears to be more rapidly fatal in women is another urgent research task.

Many long-term survivors lead more or less normal lives.

According to Dr. Hardy, "After examining the clinical and laboratory parameters on the forty-eight people we studied intensively, we found that a lot of these people are doing pretty well, even though they still have continued evidence of T-helper cell depression. Most of them are totally functional. That's an important message to get out even in itself."

Once you've survived for approximately five years, your probability of dying from AIDS levels off.

Several researchers commented on the curious fact that after five years, the cumulative probability of survival remains relatively stable at around 10 percent. Researchers were at a loss as to why this might be so; but for those of us who have survived beyond five years, it's a much-needed bit of good news.

⊠ According to the best survival data currently available, only one out of ten people with AIDS survives three or more years, and only one out of thirty-three survives five or more years. When I have told people that I'm writing a book about long-term survival based on a 9.5 percent three-or-more-years survival rate and a 3 percent five-or-more-years survival rate, most have said that they don't think such depressingly low survival figures are much to celebrate.

I have two responses. First, since people with AIDS are often told that there are no survivors at all—that AIDS is not survivable—even a 3 percent five-year survival rate is at least something to hang hope's hat upon. Secondly, the admittedly depressing survival probabilities represent the natural history of *largely untreated* AIDS. These statistics reflect the early years of AIDS, when our knowledge about managing the disease was primitive, to say the least. These figures have nowhere to go but up, as the slow but sure improvement in survival probabilities confirms.

Survival rates for full-blown AIDS are increasing for two reasons: (1) prophylaxis is preventing PCP in the first place and improvements in treatment for an actual PCP infection mean that almost no one dies from their first bout of pneumonia anymore;[14] and (2) there have undoubtedly been improvements in overall patient management.

Many mistakenly believe that AZT is responsible for most of the improvement in survival. In fact, the major reason for the dramatic improvement in survival prospects is the widespread practice of pneumocystis prophylaxis. Preventing PCP will, in a single stroke, save more lives than all the AZT in the world combined.[15]

The dramatic, clear-cut success of PCP prevention—something that ought to have been achieved years ago—makes it heartbreaking to imagine how many more long-term survivors there would undoubtedly be today if only our research priorities had been different.

Long-term survival rates could easily have been doubled and maybe even tripled or quadrupled if only the federal government had encouraged physicians to provide PCP prophylaxis to all people with AIDS.

It's worth examining in some detail the impact that the prevention of PCP might have had on survival rates, because doing so makes it abundantly clear why we must immediately focus our attention on the aggressive pursuit of ways to prevent the many other opportunistic infections that kill people with AIDS. By quantifying the impact on survival rates that a single improvement in the management of patients would have had, the case for finding ways to prevent the other OIs becomes all the more compelling.

Pneumocystis carinii pneumonia (PCP) is the number one killer of people with AIDS. According to the CDC, more than half of all deaths from AIDS are attributable to PCP.

In 1977—four years before the first case of AIDS—a placebo double-blind study[16] by Dr. Walter Hughes and colleagues proved that two double-strength Bactrim tablets a day can essentially prevent PCP from occurring in immunocompromised individuals. Thus, without spending a cent on research into the prevention of PCP, the federal government could have saved countless lives if only it had made physicians aware of the Hughes study and encouraged them to provide PCP prophylaxis to their patients who were at risk for developing PCP. At the very least, prophylaxis should have been the standard of patient care for someone with AIDS who had survived one bout of PCP.[17]

I asked a CDC statistician how many AIDS-related PCP deaths had occurred since the beginning of the epidemic. How many Americans, I asked, have needlessly suffered and died from PCP because of the lack of federal leadership on the issue of PCP prophylaxis?

The horrifying answer: As of February 20, 1989,[18] 30,534 Americans had died of AIDS-associated PCP.[19]

I repeat: 30,534 United States citizens have died from a disease that since 1977 has been essentially preventable.

Bactrim and other sulfa drugs would have prevented the overwhelming majority of these cases of PCP. The treatment breakthrough rate for people with AIDS taking Bactrim is under 10 percent per year.[20] That means that thousands who died of PCP might have survived for years because they would have avoided the bout of PCP that killed them, *if only they had been prophylaxed.*[21]

It is particularly galling to me that 16,929 of the 30,534 unnecessary PCP deaths occurred since May of 1987, the date on which I and other AIDS activists met with Dr. Anthony Fauci (the closest person we have to an AIDS czar) to ask him—no, to *beg* him—to issue interim guidelines urging physicians to prophylax those patients deemed at high risk for PCP. He steadfastly refused to issue such guidelines. His reason? No data. As a result, many more people died of PCP who didn't have to.

The main determinant of an individual's prospects for survival is the quality of the patient management he or she receives. Good patient management means prevention of opportunistic infections (through prophylaxis) and the early diagnosis and appropriate treatment of opportunistic infections that do develop.

Bluntly stated, anyone's prospects for surviving AIDS will largely depend on whether he or she has primary care at all, whether the physician is knowledgeable and experienced in caring for people with AIDS, on communication between doctor and patient, and on how aggressively the physician diagnoses, treats, and attempts to prevent opportunistic complications.

A major factor in the wide variability of survival rates among the various risk groups is access to primary care and the experience and expertise of the physician caring for an individual with AIDS. Most IV drug users with AIDS are black and Hispanic and tend to be poor. In this country, poor people who get sick are forced to depend on hospital-based care, which is generally inferior to having a private physician. This undoubtedly accounts in part for the fact that

[o]n average, black and Hispanic people with AIDS are sicker at the time of diagnosis than white PWAs and die nearly five times as rapidly.[22]

Geography also affects one's survival prospects. Physicians caring for people with AIDS in the small towns and cities of middle America rarely hear of treatment advances as quickly as their colleagues who practice in the major cities along both coasts. Jeffrey A. Beal, M.D., of Tulsa, Oklahoma, testified before Congress in 1988 that

[u]nfortunately, we [in Oklahoma] have not benefited from the knowledge and expertise gained elsewhere. The Oklahoma AIDS patient has an average five month survival as compared to the eighteen months elsewhere.[23]

If AIDS is in fact the same disease in each of us, AIDS in Tulsa should be the same as AIDS in New York City. The huge disparity in survival rates is undoubtedly due to the fact that doctors in cities with large numbers of people with AIDS simply learn how to manage their patients better.

The better your doctor, the more experience he or she has caring for PWAs, the more willing he or she is to consider unproven interventions, the better your prospects of becoming a long-term survivor. It's as simple as that.

There's no point in mincing words: We've been murdered by incompetence. Despite the expenditure of billions of dollars on federal AIDS research, we have little of value to show for it. Those who find a 9.5 percent and 3 percent three- and five-years-or-more survival rate to be depressing should understand that these rates are low because of the failure of the American government to do its job.

Thousands of Americans with AIDS would be alive today if uniform standards of proper patient management had been formulated and promoted by the federal government. The fact that the survival rates for the early years are so low is merely a measure of how our government has failed us. People diagnosed with AIDS have much brighter prospects for becoming long-term survivors thanks to PCP prophylaxis and better patient management.

The good news is that the community-based AIDS treatment research movement has made the prevention of opportunistic infections a top research priority. And as more and more lethal infections become preventable, the survival rates will soar.

⊠ Even as we wait for community-based research to find ways to keep us alive, it is time we put to rest, once and for all, the myth that no one has survived AIDS. We need to admit hope into the AIDS dialogue. Even as we take to the streets demanding radical changes in the way drugs for AIDS are tested, the epidemiology of AIDS makes it clear that, even without major treatment breakthroughs, a certain percentage have survived—and will survive—for many years beyond the current grim predictions. Analysis of survival trends and ranges justifies the hope that some percentage of those diagnosed with full-blown AIDS will, despite our disease, grow old and grumpy along with the rest of our generation.

Dr. Lemp and his colleagues have documented significant improvements in survival probability and have predicted that median survival will double from eleven months in 1981 to twenty-two months in 1993. Although every researcher I interviewed repeatedly cautioned against predicting current and future survival prospects based on extrapolations from analyses of survival from this early period, it still seems reasonable to project that these dramatic improvements in one-year median survival probability will translate into proportional dramatic improvements in three- and five-year survival probabilities. Survival rates have nowhere to go but up, based on current statistical trends and obvious improvements in patient management.

Finally, it's important to remember when examining statistics that one's individual survival prospects vary depending on a variety of interdependent factors such as gender, risk group(s), number and type of opportunistic infections, and year of diagnosis. Although the value of Dr. Rothenberg's 1987 study is limited, he did find that "the range in mortality rate was greater than threefold, depending on . . . variables."[24] Undoubtedly additional factors such as access to primary care, improvements in patient management, and potential treatment improvements will also play a large role in determining the likelihood of becoming a long-term survivor of AIDS.

It may be more useful to speak of the probabilities for survival based on specific variables than to talk about survival probability *averages*. For example, if you're a gay man whose only opportunistic infection is KS, it may be misleading and unnecessarily depressing to say that you have a 9.5 percent probability of living three or more years. In fact, evidence suggests that such a person stands a good chance of living much longer than that. The unfortunate converse, however, is that if you're a gay man with PCP, the probability is that you won't live as long as someone exactly like you demographically but whose AIDS-defining opportunistic infection is KS.

As Dr. Bernie Siegel has so eloquently pointed out in *Love, Medicine & Miracles*, statistics are useful for gaining some sense of the *probability* of a particular event. But statistics can never predict which individuals will be among the survivors and which will be among those who succumb. In the end, for each individual, it is as rational to believe he or she will be among the survivors as it is to assume that he or she won't.

NOTES

1. Most laypeople (including myself when I began to examine survival statistics) confuse "average" survival time with "median" survival time. Strictly speaking, the average survival rate would require that we add up the survival lengths for everyone diagnosed and then divide that by the number of people diagnosed. The problem with averaging is that extremes at either end—people who die on the day of their diagnosis and the handful of survivors still alive after 11 years—can skew the average. That is why epidemiologists prefer to talk about median survival. The dictionary defines median as "the middle value in a distribution, above and below which lie an equal number of values." In other words, median survival is the length of time that a majority of people with AIDS survive after diagnosis.

2. Early in 1987, Alan Kristol, Ph.D., of the New York City Department of Health, published AIDS survival data in the *American Journal of Epidemiology*. For "gay, non-IV drug-using" PWAs, he found a three-year survival rate of 16 percent and a four-year survival rate of 13 percent. For IV-drug-using, non-gay PWAs, he found a 10 percent three-year survival rate and a 5 percent four-year survival rate. Combining and averaging all PWAs, he found a 14 percent three-year survival rate and a 10 percent four-year survival rate. This study was cited in *Surviving and Thriving with AIDS*, vol. 1, which I edited and which was published by PWA Coalition (New York) in March 1987.

3. Rothenberg, Richard, M.D., et al., "Survival with the Acquired Immunodeficiency Syndrome: Experience with 5833 Cases in New York City," *The New England Journal of Medicine*, 317, no. 21 (November 19, 1987): 1297.

4. Dr. Stephen Joseph, New York City Commissioner of Health, quoted in Gina Kolata, "15% of People with AIDS Survive 5 Years," *New York Times*, November 19, 1987, sec. B.

5. Rothenberg, et al., 1297.

6. Actually, the "lost to follow-up" category is greater than 24 percent, because for reasons never made clear, the CDC didn't even attempt to do follow-up on 41 out of the original 821.

7. The low of 2.8 percent represents the worst-case scenario; it assumes that all 187 people lost to follow-up are actually dead. The 119 actual survivors out of a total of 4,073 cases reported comes to a depressing 2.8 percent three-year-or-more survival rate. If, as a best-case scenario, one assumes that all 187 people lost to follow-up are actually alive, that would mean that 306 out of 4,073 have survived AIDS for three or more years; that means the upper survival estimate is 7.5 percent.

8. Lemp, Dr. George F., P.H., Susan F. Payne, M.A., et al., "Trends in the Length of Survival for AIDS Cases in San Francisco," presented at the IVth International

Conference on AIDS, Stockholm, Sweden, 1988. See the chart entitled "Survival of AIDS Patients in San Francisco by Year of Diagnosis."

9. Dr. Stephen Joseph, quoted in Kolata.

10. Two of the four PCP survivors in Dr. Hardy's forty-eight-person study turned out to show no evidence of past infection with HIV. Dr. Hardy's arbitrary decision was to exclude these two people as "actual long-term survivors of AIDS." As she said with breathtaking bluntness, "they met the case definition for AIDS, but did not *really* have AIDS." I do not accept the arbitrary ejection of these cases from the long-term-survivor fraternity. In any event, they *are* long-term survivors of PCP. For those who agree with Dr. Hardy that the two HIV-negative long-term survivors of PCP should not be counted as long-term survivors of AIDS, the approximate number of long-term survivors of AIDS who are HIV positive and who've had PCP would be reduced from 15 to 10. But the question of HIV's relationship to AIDS raised here does not detract from the main point: There are *definitely* people with AIDS who have survived three or more years after a diagnosis of PCP.

11. One plausible explanation for the dramatic difference in survival prospects for those with KS versus those with PCP is the widely known fact that people with KS tend to have better immune function than people who get KS. KS can occur when a person has 700–800 T-helper cells, whereas PCP rarely occurs if a person has more than 200 T-helper cells.

12. See my interview with PWA long-term survivor Bruce Zachar "How Come Everyone Else Is Dying and I'm Not?" in *Surviving and Thriving with AIDS: Collected Wisdom.* Michael Callen, ed. (New York: PWA Coalition, 1988), 150–160.

13. Richard Rothenberg, M.D., et al., 1297.

14. According to Dr. W. David Hardy (author of "Prophylaxis of AIDS-Related Opportunistic Infections (OIs)," which appears in *The 1989 AIDS Clinical Review*), by 1984 "[t]herapy for first episodes of PCP [was] successful in 79–90% of patients, but this therapeutic success drops to 30–65% with recurrent episodes." According to Dr. Donald Armstrong of Memorial Sloan-Kettering, improvements in PCP treatment success depend on improving doctor/patient communications:

The 69% response rate [to Bactrim, the standard first-line therapy for PCP] represents data collected over the years. I believe that we should have a 90%+ response rate, if the doctor and the patient are communicating and listening to each other.

15. In "Prophylaxis of AIDS-Related Opportunistic Infections," *The 1989 AIDS Clinical Review,* edited by Paul Volberding, M.D., and Mark Jacobson, M.D. (New York: Marcel Dekker, 1989), Dr. W. David Hardy states bluntly:

Initial reports of the benefits of zidovudine [AZT] therapy for HIV infection indicated a decreased incidence of OIs. Optimistic authors hypothesized that zidovudine alone might obviate the need for prophylaxis of AIDS-related OIs. Unfortunately, the incidence of recurrent PCP remains little changed by zidovudine therapy without secondary prophylaxis. In an ongoing prospective study, recurrent PCP has been diagnosed in 272 of 561 (48.5%) nonprophylaxed patients receiving zidovudine over a 10-month mean follow-up period. Similarly, in a retrospective analysis, the mean time to PCP recurrence was noted to be 28.5 weeks among 16 patients receiving zidovudine compared to 35.8 weeks among 55 patients not receiving zidovudine (p = 0.21).

This last sentence is particularly shocking. Although the numbers are small, the data seem to suggest that without PCP prophylaxis, people taking AZT develop PCP *faster* than people with AIDS who aren't on AZT. (PCP recurred at 28.5 weeks for those on AZT versus 35.8 weeks for those not on AZT.) Might AZT *increase* one's risk for opportunistic infections rather than decrease it, as we are being led to believe?

Also, at a forum held at Columbia University in November 1988, one panelist indicated that out of 247 people with full-blown AIDS followed for a year and a half, 74 percent used AZT for an average of 7.8 months:

> Eighty percent of people on AZT not receiving [PCP] prophylaxis had a recurrent episode of pneumocystis. Among patients receiving aerosol pentamidine, only 5% in the 15-month period as opposed to 80% developed a recurring episode [of PCP]. This is a 16-fold reduction.

For a copy of the transcript containing this quote, send a check for $19.95 made out to CGHAP and send it to Columbia Gay Health Advocacy Project, Columbia University, 400 John Jay Hall, New York, NY 10027.

16. Hughes, W. T., Kuhn, S., Chaudhary, S., et al., "Successful chemoprophylaxis for *Pneumocystis carinii* pneumonitis," *N Engl J Med* 297 (1977): 1419–1426. See also Hughes, W. T., McNobb, P. C., Makres, T. D., et al., "Efficacy of trimethoprim and sulfamethoxazole in the prevention and treatment of *Pneumocystis carinii* pneumonitis," *J Infect Dis* 128 (1973): 607–611.

17. There is no question that people with AIDS who manage to survive their first bout of PCP are at high risk of developing subsequent bouts. According to Dr. W. David Hardy,

> PCP recurs commonly. In a retrospective report of 201 post-PCP patients not receiving [AZT] nor secondary prophylaxis, PCP recurred in 18% of patients at 6 months, 46% at 9 months, and 65% at 18 months. [Citing Rainer CA, et al., Prognosis and Natural History of Pneumocystis carinii Pneumonia: Indicators for Early and Late Survival (Abstract). International Conference on AIDS, Washington, D.C., June 1–5, 1987:THP.154.]

Despite the widely recognized fact that people with AIDS post-PCP have a great likelihood of developing subsequent bouts, as recently as June of '89, Trial 5, a federal trial led by Dr. Margaret Fischl, explicitly forbade patients who had had a bout of PCP from using any form of PCP prophylaxis. Individuals who died of PCP during this trial did not have to die.

18. When I called the CDC to find out how many people with AIDS have died of PCP, I was told that figures could only be provided through February 1989. Apparently, the CDC plans to stop collecting data about actual cause of death. Perhaps this change is due to a recognition by the federal government that it is complicit in so many unnecessary deaths and, as a consequence, wishes to frustrate future attempts

to quantify the murderous consequences of its failure to make the prevention of PCP a top priority.

19. See *AIDS Weekly Surveillance Report—United States,* published by the AIDS Program, Center for Infectious Diseases, Centers for Disease Control, February 20, 1989, and September 5, 1988. Thanks to Mary Ann Pesa of the CDC for reading me these figures.

20. Obviously, if the prophylaxis breakthrough rate is 10 percent, each year you survive you have another 10 percent chance of getting PCP despite prophylaxis. And besides, some might argue, if PCP doesn't get you, something else might. But then again, it might not!

Dr. W. David Hardy at UCLA is conducting a 200-person trial that compares Bactrim against Fansidar against aerosol pentamidine as PCP prophylaxis. Although his study has not been completed, he indicated that in the year since the study began, there have been *no* cases of PCP recurrence in those on Bactrim.

21. Today, thanks to better management, few people with AIDS die of their first bout of PCP.

According to the article by W. David Hardy, M.D., "Prophylaxis of AIDS-Related Opportunistic Infections (OIs)," from *The 1989 AIDS Clinical Review:*

Today therapy for first episodes of PCP is successful in 70–90% of patients [citations omitted], but this therapeutic success drops to 30–65% with recurrent episodes of PCP [citation omitted].

Using a 70 percent failure rate for the treatment of a second bout of PCP, 30 percent of the 198 people who were unlucky enough to have gotten another bout of PCP *despite* being on prophylaxis would have survived, resulting in another 60 people eligible for the long-term survivor sweepstakes.

22. Dalton, Harlon L., "AIDS in Blackface," *Daedalus* (1989) (special issue on AIDS), citing Sabatier, 19; V. M. Mays and S. D. Cochran, "Acquired Immunodeficiency Syndrome and Black Americans: Special Psychosocial Issues," Public Health Reports 102(2) (1987): 228; and S. R. Friedman, et al., "The AIDS Epidemic among Blacks and Hispanics," *Milbank Quarterly* 65 (suppl. 2) (1987): 477–80.

23. Testimony of Jeffrey A. Beal, M.D., Tulsa, Oklahoma, reprinted in *Therapeutic Drugs for AIDS: Development, Testing, and Availability,* transcript from Hearings before a Subcommittee of the Committee on Government Operations, House of Representatives, One Hundredth Congress, Second Session, April 28 and 29, 1988, 64.

24. Richard Rothenberg, M.D., quoted in Kolata.

WHY SOME SURVIVE

What Western Science Has to Say

THE WIZARD OF ID

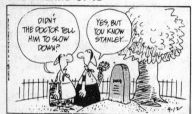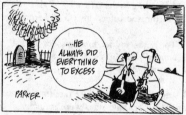

"The Wizard of Id" cartoon © 1989 by Johnny Hart. Used by permission of Johnny Hart and NAS, Inc.

▨▨▨ A few people have survived full-blown AIDS for eleven or more years. The million-dollar question that follows is, of course, why. Is there something unique about long-term survivors? Are there any biological or psychosocial factors that distinguish those who have survived? What does Western science have to say?

As a rabid rationalist who can't stomach metaphysical, New Age explanations, I found it deeply depressing to discover that science doesn't have much of value to say about—and hasn't looked very hard to discover— why some of us survive AIDS.

One of the goals of Dr. Hardy's national study was supposed to have been the "characterization" of long-term survivors. Unfortunately, the "intensive" study of a forty-eight-person subset of the 119 survivors identified by the CDC as "actually alive" consisted merely of a review of the survivors' medical records and blood tests focusing primarily on T-cell and HIV testing. The fact that a few important observations came out of even so cursory a review hints at what might have been discovered if a more extensive analysis had been performed.

Dr. Hardy acknowledged that a more extensive analysis of the laboratory and psychosocial characteristics of these long-term survivors would have been worthwhile, but defensively explained that doing so wasn't logistically feasible. Because of concerns about confidentiality, the CDC never had direct contact with any of the long-term survivors.

The CDC settled for a listing of what symptoms were present before diagnosis, at diagnosis, and at follow-up, and what each survivor's current disability status was.

Logistics aside, the major reason why Dr. Hardy and her colleagues didn't press for a more in-depth study was they didn't have detailed information on a similar group of individuals who *hadn't* survived AIDS. This lack of "controls" against which to compare what they might have found from studying the survivors made it virtually impossible to draw scientifically credible conclusions.

The trail of AIDS research is littered with dead ends and missed opportunities. I couldn't shake the feeling that once again, a tremendous opportunity had been missed. I realized during my phone interview with Dr. Hardy that despite my efforts to pose as an objective reporter intellectually interested in the phenomenon of long-term survival, I was actually a very subjective person with AIDS who urgently wanted to understand why I was still alive. As disappointment washed over me, I realized that despite the billions of dollars poured down the rat hole of federal AIDS research, the questions that truly mattered would probably never be answered. Hell, I thought, they'd probably never even be asked!

CDC AIDS researcher Dr. Richard Rothenberg is pessimistic about the prospects for an answer to the mystery of long-term AIDS survival.

A prospective study would of course be best. But even to do a good retrospective study, we'd need to review the charts of about 5,000 people with AIDS. We've also been hoisted by our own petard of confidentiality. I'm afraid we've just missed the boat on this one. The best study of long term AIDS survival hasn't been done, and probably will never be done. The logistics are insurmountable.

One hopes that the AIDS activist community will add long-term survivor studies to their long list of urgent AIDS research priorities.

▨ Perhaps the most prominent researcher willing to speculate publicly about possible mechanisms by which some people might peacefully co-exist with even full-blown AIDS is Dr. Jay Levy of the Cancer Research

Institute at the University of California at San Francisco. Recently, he has been studying the blood of long-term survivor Dan Turner to see if he can isolate, and possibly clone, some factor which might account for Dan's longevity.

In a recent article published in the *Journal of the American Medical Association,* Dr. Levy speculated that the secret of long-term survival may be the role played by CD8/suppressor T-cells. Having accepted the central tenet of HIV orthodoxy—that HIV is the primary cause of the profound immune deficiency that characterizes AIDS—Dr. Levy hypothesizes that a "selected subgroup of CD8 [T-suppressor] cell[s]" may secrete a mysterious substance ["a lymphokine whose structure is not yet defined"] which suppresses HIV infection. Dr. Levy is aggressively exploring this idea:

> The identification of the particular cells responsible is in progress. The presence of this strong antiviral activity in asymptomatic individuals offers an optimistic direction for potential antiviral therapies.[1]

Other researchers have other theories.

Dr. Jack Gorman is a biological psychologist; he explores the biological aspects of different psychiatric disorders. He is currently directing a research project called the Natural History and Progression of HIV Infection. "We call it the follow-up project, for short," he explained. "We're studying behavioral and nervous system in factors in HIV progression as a joint project between Columbia University and New York State Psychiatric Institute. We have enrolled 200 gay men and we're closing in on 200 parenteral drug users."

The study, funded for five years, has only been enrolling for a year and a half, and like other appropriately cautious scientists, Dr. Gorman emphasized that it's too early to speak with much confidence about what psychologic and biologic factors will prove to influence survival prospects. But I pressed him to speculate anyway:

> It's very hard to say scientifically why some people are long-term survivors. Some people have suggested that different strains of HIV may be involved. And of course there are cofactors.

But it is genetic influences which most intrigue him. He got very excited while explaining a recent article that discussed the role genetics may play in influencing an individual's ability to respond effectively to diseases.

It's been known for a long time that there are genetic differences in a person's response to viruses. In fact, there's a very interesting study in the *New England Journal of Medicine* that of all the different diseases in the world, the ones that people respond to differently just because of genetic differences are infectious diseases. See, one's response to an infectious disease depends on what kind of B cells you make, what kind of immunoglobulins; there's a gene for everything for all those. This study showed that in terms of genetic traits which influence families' responses to disease, the risk of dying from infectious diseases is greater within a family than the risk of dying of cancer or heart disease! It actually makes a lot of sense because as you learn about immunology you realize that every part of the immune response is controlled by a gene that codes for some protein that's an immunoglobulin. So some people who get infected with HIV may have had parents who were terrific at fighting viruses and that makes for a different prognosis.

"One more thing to blame our parents for," I joked.

▨ Dr. Hardy, who has recently left the CDC for greener pastures, expressed the hope that Western science would pursue an explanation for the phenomenon of long-term AIDS survival. "There's some reason why these people have survived," she asserted. "The answer's there. It's just a matter of finding it."

But it is unclear whether much is being done at the federal level to find answers. Testifying before the President's Commission on HIV, Dr. Larry Siegel, a Key West, Florida, physician whose area of expertise is the interrelationship of AIDS and chemical dependency, urged the immediate, intensive study of long-term survivors. Unfortunately, I can find nothing in the final commission report that recommends such a study.

It seems clear that we cannot rely on federal research to solve the mystery of long-term survival. And it is unclear to what extent federally funded natural history studies are collecting the kind of detailed information that might permit researchers at some future date to speak with confidence about what factors contribute to long-term survival. In the best of circumstances, it will be many, many years before enough time has lapsed to permit reliable conclusions to be drawn. And given the budget deficit, competition for funding among advocates for research into other diseases, and the low value placed by American society on the lives of those affected by AIDS, there is no guarantee of public support for continued funding of these expensive, labor-intensive, prospective natural history studies.

The most exciting work being done on the psychologic and biologic aspects of long-term AIDS survival is the work of Dr. George Solomon and Dr. Lydia Temoshok (which will be discussed below). Their work has been considered so controversial that federal support for it has only recently been granted. According to Dr. Solomon,

> Our long-term AIDS survivors study was paid for with private money from Norman Cousins and the Task Force on Psychoneuroimmunology at UCLA. If you're doing anything innovative, let's face it, you'll need private money. At first we couldn't get any money. The National Institute of Mental Health wouldn't pay for any lab work, so we couldn't get any immune studies. And National Institute of Health wouldn't pay for any psychological studies. We just couldn't get any money. It was awful. It's a much better situation now than it had been. Now NIMH will pay for lab studies.

Dr. George Lemp, the San Francisco epidemiologist who is closely monitoring survival trends, joined the unanimous chorus of researchers I interviewed who are frustrated that there aren't more and better studies of the phenomenon of long-term AIDS survival.

> It's obviously important to study long-term survivors. They may provide clues. And I'm not satisfied with the number of studies that are going on about long-term survival and survival in general. There aren't that many articles on survival, or on what increases survival. Or [survival] in relation to other factors. There have always been a small number of people looking at survival, which I always thought was important. I don't know why there seems to be a bias against studying AIDS survival. Maybe people don't want to study something that appears to be depressing or maybe people assume that everyone is dying. The majority of studies have focused on progression from infection with HIV to AIDS and have not focused on persons who already have AIDS. But I think studying long term survival is important.

⊠ Most people believe that conquering AIDS will require new therapies. But for those familiar with the sad saga of AIDS treatment research, it doesn't seem likely that the cure for AIDS will come anytime soon. Therefore there is great interest among people with AIDS in those areas where self-intervention might make some difference.

Common wisdom available on the PWA grapevine counsels the newly diagnosed PWA to "listen to your body." This advice is a mushy blend of New Age slogans and grandma's commonsensical advice. Fortunately, for those of us looking for some rational reason to believe that attitude can make a difference in our survival prospects, a new field of research entirely devoted to exploring the mind/body connection has been generating a number of exciting hypotheses which seem potentially applicable to designing a long-term survival strategy for AIDS.

In 1964, George F. Solomon, M.D., launched a new field of research known by the daunting name of "psychoneuroimmunology." The name was chosen in part to give scientific legitimacy to the study of what has been referred to as the mind/body connection. Dr. Solomon is infectiously enthusiastic about the knowledge generated by psychoneuroimmunology in its brief history. During the past three decades, Dr. Solomon and his fellow psychoneuroimmunologists have generated a number of fascinating "postulates" which, in plain English, propose that thoughts and emotions profoundly affect the course of a disease by marshalling or impairing the complex immune responses of the body.

To be more reductive than Dr. Solomon and his colleagues would probably be comfortable with, psychoneuroimmunology may someday be able to explain in empiric terms just what "having the right attitude" might mean and how precisely it might contribute to health.

Because AIDS is a disease of immune regulation, it presents a unique opportunity for psychoneuroimmunology to test its mettle. If research can prove that long-term survivors have some unique coping style, such a finding would go a long way toward confirming many of the postulates of psychoneuroimmunology and, more importantly, would suggest ways to extend life while we wait for a cure.

If one asked laboratory scientists and AIDS researchers whether attitude affects survival, most would probably dismiss the notion as unscientific. But these are often the same scientists who refuse to consider clinical trial data which was not gathered as the result of placebo double-blind trials. Psychoneuroimmunology is merely an extension of the implications contained in the notion of placebo effects.

A condescending dictionary definition[2] of placebo inadvertently captures allopathic medicine's contempt for the idea that attitude might affect the course of a disease. A placebo is defined as "a substance containing no medication and given *merely to humor a patient.*" (Emphasis added.)

Someone whose symptoms actually, observably, objectively disappear while taking a sugar pill may be "humoring" him- or herself, but the placebo effect nevertheless proves that *believing* in the possibility of healing—and *believing* that one is doing something to bring it about—often has beneficial effects. It isn't necessary to deny that the ultimate solution to AIDS will require allopathic drugs to admit that hope might improve survival probabilities.

It is interesting to make explicit the reasons behind Western science's fanatic adherence to the gold standard of placebo, double-blind clinical trials. "Double-blind" means that neither the physician nor the patient knows whether a particular patient is getting the experimental drug or a sugar pill. The reason why physicians aren't supposed to know comes from the recognition that they might treat patients receiving drug differently, i.e., better than, patients receiving a sugar pill. Doctors generally recoil from the suggestion that how they treat their patients—the emotional messages they send—may affect the course of a patient's illness. But science's insistence on double-blinding implicitly recognizes that this phenomenon occurs.[3]

The reason why patients in clinical trials aren't supposed to know whether they're receiving drug or placebo is precisely because studies have proven that such knowledge affects the patient's condition. The fact that people on placebo often improve—sometimes doing even better than people receiving medication—compels an acknowledgment that attitude can affect healing.[4]

▨ For those of us eager for Western science to come up with some answers as to why some people have survived AIDS, our best hope is probably the preliminary, largely descriptive work of Dr. Solomon, Lydia Temoshok, Ph.D., and their colleagues.

Dr. Solomon, Dr. Temoshok, and others have completed a study on eighteen long-term "AIDS" survivors. (Not all their subjects were long-term survivors of full-blown AIDS; several "only" had AIDS-Related Complex.)

In addition to extensive blood work, the researchers monitored survivors for skin conductance, respiration, heart rate, and finger temperature while the subjects described their past week's experience of anger, happiness, fear, and love.

Dr. Solomon refers to this study as "impressionistic," and during our several phone interviews repeatedly cautioned against overinterpretating results based on such a small number of subjects. Dr. Temoshok is even more cautious about drawing conclusions on the basis of their study. Despite their cautions, both were willing to say that their study confirmed that "positive coping was positively correlated with a variety of immune functions." ("Positive coping" is fancy psychoneuroimmunological argot for "having the right attitude.")

In designing their study, Dr. Solomon's group did something radical in its simplicity: They asked a group of five long-term survivors to act as "consultants" and to describe the factors which they felt had contributed to their longevity. Using the survivors' self-assessments, Drs. Temoshok and Solomon designed study questionnaires. (To avoid bias, the five "consultants" were not part of the eighteen-person group whose data was analyzed.)

After comparing the factors identified by the consultants with reports from survivors of other life-threatening diseases, the Solomon group hypothesized a number of characteristics that might distinguish long-term survivors of AIDS. Paraphrased and condensed, they proposed that:

1. Survivors are realistic about the seriousness of their condition without being fatalistic. They refuse to believe AIDS is an "automatic death sentence."

2. Survivors are willing to take responsibility for their own healing and to make major life-style adjustments to "accommodate disease in an adaptive way." Survivors believe that physical fitness and exercise contribute to healing and believe that their "personalized means of active coping" can have "beneficial health effects."

3. Survivors tend to have extraordinary relationships with their healthcare providers. Survivors spoke of a healing partnership with their healthcare providers, and were neither passively compliant nor defiant.

4. Survivors are passionately committed to living and have a sense of "meaningfulness and purpose in life," of "unmet goals." Often the diagnosis itself enables them to find "new meaning" to life.

5. Survivors tend to have faced and to have overcome past life crises.

6. Meeting and talking with other people with AIDS in a supportive environment, especially shortly after their own diagnosis, was deemed important. Being "altruistically involved" with other people with AIDS— being self-concerned without being exclusively self-involved—was considered beneficial by survivors.

7. Survivors are assertive and able to communicate openly, including the ability to say no. Survivors "nurture" themselves and are "sensitive to their body and its needs."

This list of traits jived with my own sense of the characteristics shared by the long-term survivors I have known. But Dr. Solomon apparently has *laboratory* evidence which, he said, "essentially confirmed" that these traits can improve immune function. Dr. Temoshok indicated that "being able to say no to unwanted favors was important across a number of immune variables."

Like other PWAs, I spend much of my time translating the mumbo jumbo of experts into plain English. "Important across a number of immune variables" didn't mean much to me.

"Are you saying," I asked, "that the 'ability to say no' was a predictive characteristic of long-term survivors?"

But she steadfastly refused to give me a simple yes or no. Instead, she used the complicated question of whether exercise improves immune function to explain why, given the inconclusive nature of the data, she was unwilling to advise PWAs about what to do:

> Our long-term survivor study found that exercising more regularly seemed to be involved with more natural killer cell production. But is it good or bad for people with AIDS to have higher natural killer cell activity? We don't know. Based on our small study, I would *never* advocate that people with AIDS should go out and moderately exercise. Increased natural killer cell activity may be maladaptive. We simply don't know what the relationship is. So I'm not advocating interventions one way or the other. A lot of these interventions are potentially powerful and unless you know what you're doing, you may paradoxically do something that may not be in the best interest of a particular person's physiologic adaptations to coping with this disease.

To further confuse matters, Dr. Solomon confessed that although

> positive coping was positively correlated with a variety of immune functions, everything came out exactly the opposite in a similar study of people with AIDS-Related Complex. I can't really account for it. In people with ARC, *more* distress correlated with better immune function and vice versa—just the opposite of the long term survivors.

When I asked what might explain the paradox that emotional distress appeared to be correlated with improved immune response in people with ARC whereas *resolving* emotional distress was correlated with improved immune function in people with full-blown AIDS, Dr. Solomon speculated that

> there's some work to suggest that the immunopathology is quite different between ARC and AIDS, since early on, the defect is the overactivation of the immune system which results in a failure to return to baseline. So there is never the development of a store of immune memory cells and this, in turn, ultimately leads to the severe immunodeficiency we call AIDS. So the impact of psychoso-

cial events on a phase of an overstimulated immune system versus a shot system, let us say, may be different. But we also have some more immune studies cooking that we haven't fully tabulated on this ARC sample.

He seemed genuinely puzzled and intrigued about the finding:

Everything looked so neat until the ARC data did not confirm the AIDS data. The AIDS data we have is *very* much in line with the impressionistic sense we had.

Dr. Solomon hinted that his published report on this study would contain a number of intriguing correlations between attitude and immune improvement. Until the results are published, however, the closest thing to advice for long-term survivors that I could extract from my conversations with Drs. Solomon and Temoshok was the following generalization by Dr. Temoshok:

It's probably safe to say that *dis*-stress is bad for you. Distress indicates a failure of coping. In other words, stress itself is neither good nor bad. It's how we deal with it.

She supported the holistic principle that it is important to listen to one's own body, and one's thoughts and emotions:

Listen to your body and to your mind as to how you're feeling. For example, if you're running and your body doesn't feel good, stop running. Or if you find yourself getting mad at someone a lot, maybe that isn't such a good person to hang around with. Better to hang around with people who make you feel better. Or if your job is not providing a sense of meaning but is just providing hassles, that may be something to question. In other words, pay attention to all of your symptoms, whether they're physiological or psychological. If you're feeling distressed, those feelings are telling you something; listen to them. It's not *bad* to have those feelings; feelings are signals that something is wrong in your environment, and the idea is to do something to change whatever is wrong. So that's all I would say.

My conversations with Drs. Solomon and Temoshok confirmed my own suspicions that each person's healing strategy would be individualized. One man's stress is another man's distress. For me, sugar is a reason to live; for the holistically inclined who believe a "proper" diet is the basis of all healing, my commitment to Classic Coke is anathema.

But I worried that "listen to your own body" was too glib of a generalization to be useful. I asked Dr. Temoshok if she was suggesting that one's attitude was all that mattered—that determining whether, say, sugar was a good thing or a bad thing for someone with AIDS would depend primarily on whether one *believed* sugar was good or bad.

She bristled at the oversimplification and said that it was precisely such misrepresentations of psychoneuroimmunology that trouble her:

> A common and dangerous misconception is that we're saying that if you're sick, you must have a bad attitude and that getting well is a simple matter of having the "right" attitude. That's wrong, dead wrong. It is very negative for anyone who has a disease to have the feeling that he or she is to blame for it because of his or her attitude, and that if only he or she had the "right attitude," the disease would miraculously go away.

She ended by giving me the kind of advice that my grandmother might have given me:

> I think there are complicated relationships between thoughts and emotions and the immune response to distress. Distress indicates a failure of coping and acts as a warning to take control and help your body to adapt both psychologically and physiologically to its environment. That has to be positive. I would, myself, not want to use the words "right attitude," because it gets people thinking, "Well, I'm dying of AIDS so therefore I must have the wrong attitude and therefore it's my fault." And then you get into blaming, which doesn't help anyone. I think I'd rather be descriptive about things— just say that of the people who live the longest, they happen to have those feelings.

Dr. Solomon remains optimistic about the ability of psychoneuroimmunology to crack the mystery of why some of us have survived AIDS beyond expectations. While the search goes on, he felt it was important to keep challenging the myth that AIDS is invariably fatal.

> People have been extrapolating the exponential curve of death and then concluding that everyone who's HIV positive is going to die. Well, I don't believe it. In the first place, we know there's enormous variability with AIDS. Since survival is possible, isn't there a likelihood that one can shift these curves, that you can help people live longer, more healthy lives? The obsession in the media and at the professional level with AIDS being an automatic death sentence feeds upon itself. Hopelessness and helplessness are the very worst emotions. Hopelessness is the component of depression which is the most malignant to the immune system. We knew that way before AIDS.

I told Dr. Solomon that the myth of 100 percent mortality made me angry. He responded:

> Your anger is *terrific!* Anger is protective. It's the nice guys that go down—the ones who are sweetly compliant and cooperative with their doctors. Its the sons-of-bitches, the ones who kick and scream and yell who do better. The doctors don't like them so much, but they do better. My advice: Stay angry!

Dr. Temoshok shared her colleague's optimism that psychoneuroimmunology might help crack the mystery of long-term AIDS survival. But she believed much more research would be needed. She also felt that opinions about the inevitability of death from AIDS were changing:

> Because of AZT and other medications, the perception of AIDS as being universally fatal is changing to one of a chronic disease. I think that's good. Since '83, we've been arguing that you can't say it's 100 percent fatal if there are still people who are alive and doing well. But I don't think they're coming around because they think that psychological things make a difference. I think they're coming around because they think that medical science is going to do something about AIDS. I think the reception by the straight biomedical establishment for the idea of psychoneuroimmunological research into HIV is really very mixed.

Indeed, many scientists remain skeptical about the findings of psychoneuroimmunology. For instance, when I asked San Francisco AIDS researcher Dr. George Lemp whether he thought there was a survival personality, or whether he thought that behavior and attitude can actually impact on survival, he voiced the common opinion of many researchers:

> Studies have shown that attitudes can affect things somewhat, but I think it's a minor part of the picture. The more important factors are what diagnoses a person has, what type of treatments they get and how they care for themselves health-wise, nutritionally, etc. People who live longer may have a good attitude, but that may be a false association. It's mainly a person's individual ability to respond to an infection. Also, there's some luck involved.

New York AIDS researcher Dr. Jack Gorman shared some of Dr. Lemp's skepticism:

> There's an open question in HIV research and in all of cancer and infectious disease research about whether things like stress, mood, and anxiety are bad for the immune system and therefore whether they might make people who get

illnesses do less well. I'm not a psychoneuroimmunologist, though I think they raise some interesting questions. There's solid science to support the idea that the central nervous system has influence over the immune system and vice versa. That part is very hard scientifically. There are nerve cells in lymph glands; and lymphocytes have receptors for neurotransmitters; and when experimental animals have an immune response, the hypothalamus in the brain starts firing. So all of that is absolutely true. What is very much less clear is whether or not depressed people get cancer more often, or if depressed people with HIV go on to get sick faster. In fact, I must tell you that so far, preliminary evidence from our study argues *against* that being the case. But, again, I can't say for sure. A lot of people would like to believe this, but so far, the scientific studies, to my mind, are not proving it. On the other hand, nobody's *disproved* it. But there's no hard proof of it—yet.

Unfortunately, much of the data on the influence of attitude on long-term survival is "soft," inconclusive, and/or contradictory. Even Bernie Siegel, evangelist of hope for many people with AIDS and other potentially terminal conditions, has been accused of ignoring or downplaying data that doesn't support his message that hope can make a difference in one's survival prospects. Some of the data he is accused of ignoring concerns a comparison of the survival times for members of the Exceptional Cancer Patients (ECaP) support group, which Dr. Siegel founded, with those who didn't participate in the support group.

A recent hostile profile of Siegel which appeared in *New York* magazine questioned whether attitude actually increases one's prospects for long-term survival:

> How valuable is ECaP? An article summarizing the results appeared in *The Journal of Chronic Diseases* in 1984. The study was conducted among 34 women with breast cancer who had attended ECaP. The purpose was to assess whether such a support group had any impact on the length of survival, as compared with patients who did not attend a group. The conclusion was that participating in ECAP had *no measurable positive impact,* no matter how long the patient attended groups. On the other hand, such a small sample is far from conclusive.[5] [emphasis added]

☒ I ended my interviews intrigued, but still longing for more conclusive evidence. As desirable as it would be to have controlled, prospective studies on large numbers of people with AIDS in order to more rigorously characterize what factors distinguish long-term survivors, it doesn't seem likely that such studies will ever be done. That means that the best evidence available is descriptive and impressionistic and will come from long-term survivors themselves.

NOTES

1. Levy, Jay A., M.D., "Human Immunodeficiency Viruses and the Pathogenesis of AIDS," from State of the Art/Review, edited by Don Risenberg, M.D., Senior Editor, *JAMA*, 261, no. 20 (May 26, 1989): 2997–3006.

2. *The American Heritage Dictionary of the English Language*, William Morris, ed. (Boston: Houghton Mifflin, 1978).

3. Although never discussed in polite company, the fact that physicians quickly figured out who was getting AZT and who was not during the multicenter trial which led to the disastrous, hasty approval of AZT may account for the fact that a disproportionate number died in the placebo arms of the trial. For a devastating critique of the AZT multicenter trial, see Sonnabend, J. A., "Review of AZT multicenter trial data obtained under the Freedom of Information Act by Project Inform and ACT-UP," in *AIDS Forum*, 1, no. 1 (January 1989): 9.

4. In recent diatribes stridently denouncing the use of placebos in AIDS clinical trials, there has been no acknowledgment of Chinese medicine's long-standing ethical objection to blinding of therapeutic trials. If one admits that *believing* that something will work can help it to do so, it is inherently unethical to deny someone precise knowledge of what they're being asked to take or do.

5. Schwartz, Tony, "Doctor Love: Best-Seller Bernie Siegel and His Controversial Theories of Self-Healing," *New York* (June 12, 1989): 40.

THE PROPAGANDA OF
HOPELESSNESS

▨▨▨ The children's rhyme is wrong: Just like sticks and stones, words *can* harm us. Knowing firsthand the consequences of the way people talk about AIDS, I have tried to trace the source of the gloom and doom. Who started the malicious lie that everyone dies of AIDS, and how is the lie maintained? Is the media to blame? The doctors? The government? AIDS activists?

The trail leads inevitably to the media. When virtually every newspaper and magazine article, every radio and television broadcast about AIDS explicitly or implicitly reinforces the message that AIDS is invariably fatal, the media clearly bears enormous responsibility for the public's perception of AIDS as an automatic death sentence.

In an attempt to track down the source of the fatalism that pervades media reports about AIDS, I interviewed many of the top AIDS reporters in the United States: Bruce Lambert of the *New York Times*, Marilyn Chase of the *Wall Street Journal*, Heidi Evans of the New York *Daily News*, Laurie Garrett (formerly with National Public Radio and now with *New York Newsday*), Catherine Woodard of *New York Newsday*, Victor Zonana of the *Los Angeles Times*, Randy Shilts of the *San Francisco Chronicle*, and Jim Bunn, formerly with KPIX-TV in San Francisco. Referred to by one of their number as the "AIDS pack," these journalists represent the cream of the crop and are highly regarded by federal researchers and AIDS activists alike. I asked them if they felt that AIDS reporting was generally fatalistic and why they thought that might be so.

Bruce Lambert, who covers AIDS for the *New York Times*, acknowledged that reporters foment fatalism:

I'm probably guilty of almost always putting in the really devastating sense about AIDS, and I suspect many other reporters are too. We talk about the "deadly epidemic" and the "tragic toll." We say, "We've already had our first Vietnam and now we're working on our second one." Projections always focus on death. Yes, 60,000 Americans have been killed by this thing; there's no getting around that. But reporters have to be careful—and we're probably not careful enough—to make it clear that not necessarily everybody dies of AIDS.

Articles on long-term survival are so rare that the chance of their making a dent in the public's conceptualization of AIDS as "invariably fatal" is slim. Bruce Lambert admitted, "I know that back in 1987, the *Times* did one story on long-term survival. But in terms of ongoing reporting of that, it probably hasn't been repeated often enough."

The few stories about long-term AIDS survival that *have* appeared have generally been marred by contempt for those who cling to the hope of long-term survival.

As if to say "don't believe what you're about to read," an editor for the *Cedar Rapids Gazette* penned the following introduction to an Associated Press profile of long-term survivors that ran in December 1989:

> *While AIDS remains inevitably fatal*, its diagnosis is not an immediate death sentence. One study found almost 10 percent of people with AIDS survived at least three years after diagnosis. As doctors learn more about AIDS and develop new drugs, they expect the number of "survivors" to grow. Here are sketches of three men living with AIDS. [emphasis added][1]

The editor underscores his contempt for the concept of an AIDS survivor by putting the word "survivors" in quotes, as if to say "of course, they're not *really* going to survive AIDS, but we'll call them survivors just to humor them."

In another glaring example of mean-spirited writing about the phenomenon of long-term survival, a *Time* magazine article[2] put the most negative spin possible on the subject. The pessimism that riddles this article is achieved as much by what is not mentioned as by what is. For example, the *Time* article referred only to Dr. Hardy's study, which found a depressing 2 to 5 percent long-term survival rate; the writers deliberately[3] failed to even mention Dr. Rothenberg's study, which had found a more optimistic 15.2 percent five-year survival rate.

Referring to the 2 to 5 percent three-year survival estimate, they wrote: "Such slender evidence is often taken as proof by desperate members of the homosexual community that they can overcome AIDS." By what logic can the existence of hundreds of survivors, some of whom have survived for more than five years, be considered "slender" proof that AIDS can be "overcome"? The existence of a single survivor proves that

AIDS can be—and has been—survived well beyond the dire predictions. The only desperation I detect is that of reporters who are perhaps nervous that they may not have been correct when they reported that there were no known survivors!

The article ends by belittling the "glimmer of hope amid the devastation being wrought by AIDS"—a "glimmer" the authors had every intention of extinguishing.

As these examples illustrate, an editor's or a reporter's choice of words can subtly, or sometimes *not* so subtly, emphasize doom. Reading from an Associated Press wire story[4], Lambert pointed out a good example of this:

> The wire story says: "A simple ten-minute test expected to be licensed later this year uses colors to tell patients if they are infected with the AIDS virus— white for health and blue for medical tragedy." Well, I mean, that's kind of loading it with emotional connotations. They could simply say "white for uninfected and blue for infected." But "medical tragedy"?

Lambert said that he has learned to choose his words carefully.

> In the early years of the epidemic, I undoubtedly wrote "often fatal" or "usually fatal" or words to that effect, but less so in the past year or so because the facts have changed. There are clearly long-term survivors and there are those who are living long and living better even if they do go into a terminal stage. I choose adjectives and adverbs that are less than absolute, because to do otherwise just wouldn't be correct.
>
> Just last week, an editor called me. He had an AIDS story he was editing from somebody else and wanted to put a line in. He asked, "What's our catch phrase? What do we say? Is it a terminal illness?" And I said, "Well, now, you really can't say that. There *are* some long-term survivors. You can say that it's 'often fatal,' or 'usually fatal'—but even 'usually' is a little strong and I wouldn't want to say that." I told him that people are living longer and better.

Reporters do not write in a vacuum. They are subject to forces beyond their individual control: subtle and not-so-subtle pressure to tow the party line; generally low, and rapidly lowering, journalistic standards; the meddling of editors and publishers; the tendency toward compression and generalization; and the limitations of space and airtime. All these factors encourage the tone of fatalism that characterizes most AIDS reporting and affects what ends up in print.

But even when *reporters* choose their words carefully, editors have the final say. *Wall Street Journal* reporter Marilyn Chase, who is responsible for some of the best AIDS reporting around, recalled an instance that illustrates the sensitive journalist's dilemma.

> In the boilerplate paragraph in which we always describe the illness, in a sentence in which I would have preferred to say that "AIDS is a lethal virus for which no cure had been found," someone who was editing this particular piece substituted the phrase "it is invariably fatal" as a flat statement. I don't think I challenged the substitution, because it either escaped my notice or was added later in the editing process. A few days after the piece ran, I received a call and a letter. The letter was *very* strong and it was from a person with AIDS who said to me, "How do you feel when you tear away people's hope? Please don't be comforted by the thought that you were only doing your job." It was *very* strong and unhappy; it left no quarter for any sort of rationalization or any sort of comforting thoughts that it couldn't have been helped. It wasn't from someone whose name was known to me and I think that that made it, if anything, more painful, because it was a private individual and it was really a deeply personal *cri de coeur* of agony and it made me feel helpless.

But, she warned, it would be simplistic, and incorrect, to conclude that the fatalism is solely the result of mean-spirited editors or newspaper policies dictating how the mortality of AIDS is described:

> I certainly don't mean to suggest that it's *Wall Street Journal* policy to always describe AIDS as invariably fatal. I want to be real clear that in my experience, differences over language have not been the result of an editorial policy. They've been matters of individual *taste*, and reasonable people will reach different conclusions about how best to accurately describe a situation.

The fatalism that pervades AIDS reportage is also reinforced by headlines and photographs. For example, a recent *New York Post* cover story[5] was headlined in two-and-a-half-inch letters: *"DYING AIDS DOC'S AGONY."* Preceding "AIDS" by the gerund "DYING" is intentionally redundant for emphasis, inasmuch as every "AIDS victim" is presented in the media as merely, inevitably, dying. Throughout the brief article, "dying" and its cousin "deadly" are used descriptively five times.

This *Post* story featured two photos of beautiful, perfectly healthy-looking Dr. Veronica Prego. In neither photo did Dr. Prego display anything like the wasted, disfigured appearance associated with the image of all people with AIDS in the public's imagination. To compensate, reporter Lucette Lagnado had to strain to pathologize Dr. Prego with prose: "She seemed more frail than just five months ago. . . . There were faint sores around her mouth—an outward sign of the painful infection associated with AIDS. . . ." *The* painful infection associated with AIDS? Which one? The precise nature of "the infection associated with AIDS" is, of course, never specified—presumably to allow the reader's imagination to run wild.

I clearly recall a painful experience I had with a photographer early in the AIDS epidemic. This photographer, who went on to win a number of awards for his photographs of people with AIDS, made an appointment to photograph me for a *Newsweek* story. When he arrived, he looked me over and then snorted contemptuously: "Where are your lesions? I need someone with lesions!" This was before I had developed KS, and when I told him I didn't have lesions, he stormed out, cursing the writer who had given the photo editor my number.

Jane Rosett, a free-lance photographer whose powerful portraits of people living with AIDS have appeared in the lesbian and gay press as well as in such mainstream publications as *Paris Match, Time, Life,* and the *New York Times,* pointed out how resistance to the very notion of long-term AIDS survival gets expressed in the images chosen by photo editors. She was asked to provide photos of long-term survivors for an article that appeared in a major weekly newspaper:

> The photo editor was very resistant to running portraits I had submitted because the people were "too healthy-looking." Basically, as far as the editor was concerned, the people I presented didn't have enough lesions.

When she submitted a portrait of two long-term survivors kissing, the editor rejected the photo, saying, "They look so normal, it could be just any gay couple."

"That was the point of the photo," she explained. "And,

> this is the attitude I've encountered over the past five years. AIDS means death to these people and when you challenge them with the idea of people *not* dying, they respond by raising all sorts of questions about whether the person actually has AIDS, whether they're lying or they've been misdiagnosed. The whole concept of a long-term survivor is threatening to most photo editors. It's just not visual enough.

Doomsday reportage is not, of course, limited to newspapers and magazines. Television AIDS reporting is at least as pathetic. Wondering whether I might not be exaggerating the media's role in maintaining a sense of helplessness and fatalism, I took a break from writing this chapter. While ironing shirts, I absently flipped through the TV channels and landed on a syndicated newsmagazine show called "This Evening." A segment about AIDS on campus introduced "Joshua," a handsome, articulate young man shown lecturing fellow college students about the horrors of AIDS. During the brief segment, we learn that Joshua is merely HIV antibody positive. No AIDS- or ARC-defining opportunistic infections are ever mentioned and no symptoms are ever described. In grave tones, the announcer describes Joshua as someone who was infected at the age of twenty through a sexual contact; pausing ever so briefly for dramatic effect, she states: "Doctors have told him that he probably has less than a year to live." The segment ends with Joshua confirming virtually every detail of an inevitably fatal "conveyor belt" conceptualization of AIDS. He says that his only hope is for a swift, painless death; but squaring his jaw bravely, he says that he *knows* that dying of AIDS is usually a long, slow process. (No doubt he gets this knowledge from the media.)

Although bad, irresponsible, simplistic AIDS reporting predominates, there is, of course, good, responsible, nuanced work. While legions of indifferent, thoughtless journalists crank out endless apocalyptic AIDS drivel, a handful of serious, sensitive reporters agonize over their choice of adjectives and adverbs, aware of the impact words can have on people with AIDS.

New York Newsday reporter Laurie Garrett put it this way:

> Look, every step of the way in this disease, there's been a learning curve for every journalist who's been covering it that's got any sensitivity at all. And part of that learning curve is realizing how words affect the people who read them. There's the words that cause hysteria in the general public or lead to backlash, and then there are words that are issues of sensitivity for people who are at risk or who in fact have AIDS.

I consider the reporters I interviewed for this chapter to be sensitive, caring people. Many of them have gotten to know and care about people with AIDS. But I suspected that they might unconsciously be allowing their own private sense of doom about AIDS to work its way into their writing. To test my suspicion, I decided to find out whether they were aware that nearly one out of every ten people with AIDS was surviving three or more years.

In a delicious exercise in table-turning, I asked them to state for the record their sense of the current survival probabilities for people with AIDS, and to offer an educated guess about the longest recorded survival of a person with AIDS. Many protested that when writing a story, they would always consult the latest statistics. All were correctly aware that at any given time roughly half of all reported cases have died. But I pressed my point. I felt that as reporters who cover AIDS on a daily basis, they should *know* what it had taken me months of research to uncover.

"For someone diagnosed with AIDS this afternoon, how long, on average," I asked, "would they be expected to live? And what is the longest AIDS survival time recorded in the medical literature?"

Only one of the top reporters I interviewed—reporters who write almost exclusively about AIDS—had an accurate sense of current survival probabilities. And all were startled to learn that CDC figures indicate that several PWAs are still alive and kicking more than a decade after being diagnosed with AIDS.

I asked Catherine Woodard, who covers AIDS for *New York Newsday*, if she could explain why she and other AIDS reporters hadn't discovered for themselves that, whether accurate or not, 14.2 percent of those diagnosed with AIDS in New York City are currently listed in official statistics as having survived five or more years. After a long pause, she bluntly responded:

> You mean, other than sloppy journalism? No, I can't. I'm sure it has to do with a lot of the points you'll be making. We don't tend to write about good news. We give lip service to *living with* AIDS, but when you think about it, the thrust of the coverage is still "AIDS as a deadly disease." It's just sloppy journalism on all of our parts. See, we use the statistics all the time for different things, when it's convenient. That information is readily available, but . . .

Her ellipses said it all.

I pointed out to her that statistics focusing on the number of people *living* with AIDS are not, in fact, readily available. The monthly AIDS update published by the New York City Health Department lists *deaths* by year of diagnosis. Anyone who cares to know how many people are still listed as being alive has to take the ten minutes necessary to perform some human calculus—converting the percentage of known dead to the actual number of those who died, then subtracting it from the total number of cases reported—to arrive at the number still listed as alive.[6]

But would it be asking too much, I asked, for a reporter whose main beat is AIDS to take the ten minutes to convert the statistics? Woodard explained that:

> One of the problems about daily journalism in particular is that nuances are often the first things to get lost—like not taking the extra ten minutes to work out the percentage of people alive. Particularly if you write for a paper where

your length is gonna be short and you can only make a couple of points, a lot of the things which you consider nuances get lost regularly. Now, if you're responsible about it, you find some way to package those elsewhere.

▨ Journalists, of course, justify their doomsday presentation of AIDS by claiming that they only pass along what the medical experts are saying. Virtually every reporter I interviewed acknowledged that medical and government experts had communicated implicitly, and often explicitly, that everyone who gets AIDS will die of it.

When I asked Garrett whether she had ever interviewed an AIDS expert who spoke in apocalyptic terms about the inevitability of death from AIDS, she responded:

Oh, yes! From the highest levels of AIDS research down to physicians in the trenches. And all over the world.

Heidi Evans of the New York *Daily News* has had the same experience:

I think there was a sense until very recently that AIDS was invariably fatal, even though they didn't always say it explicitly. I remember when I first started to report on this, experts would say "invariably fatal." And even if they didn't say it, there was a tacit understanding: There is no cure for this, there is no vaccine, and it's still this tremendously puzzling and mysterious virus that they felt defeated by.

Community physicians must bear responsibility for their role in maintaining the myth that no one has survived AIDS. In the early days of AIDS, it must have seemed to the frontline physicians that everyone *did* die. All the clinicians I interviewed confessed that their sense of AIDS is still overwhelmingly one of death. They spoke heartbreakingly of the helplessness they feel as physicians, unable to alter the course of a disease. It is as if *their* capacity for hope has atrophied after years of having little to offer while patient after patient died.

Physicians' resistance to the very idea of long-term survival is deeply entrenched and is often expressed as barely concealed *suspicions* or outright accusations of fraud whenever they encounter a long-term survivor. For instance, when I speak publicly and say that I've interviewed nearly three dozen long-term survivors, physicians present will often blurt out— just a bit too quickly—"They all only have KS, right?" "Only" KS? Many people with AIDS *die* from KS. Why should surviving AIDS-related KS be seen as not so extraordinary?

I inform these skeptics that, no, not all long-term survivors have "only" KS; I *have* interviewed long-term survivors of PCP. "*Bronchoscopy-proven PCP?*" they inquire, as if personally threatened by the assertion that people have survived, and are surviving, full-blown AIDS.

▨ Community doctors, faced with the daunting task of keeping their patients alive on a day-to-day basis, have had their hopelessness reinforced by official pronouncements that contained a sense of 100 percent mortality. For example, a brochure sent to every American household by then Surgeon General C. Everett Koop stated that

> [a]bout half . . . of persons known to have AIDS in the United States to date . . . have died of the disease. Since there is no cure, the others are expected to also eventually die from their disease.[7]

Since AIDS stories are often little more than rewritten government press releases, it is not surprising that the sense of fatalism that has paralyzed the federal response has been uncritically transmitted to—and through—the press.

The two federal officials in charge of AIDS treatment research have recently and bluntly admitted that AIDS fatalism has been pervasive among government researchers. The highest-ranking government AIDS scientist,[8] Dr. Anthony Fauci, explicitly acknowledged the general federal perception that everyone with AIDS would eventually die of it:

> Fauci said the [recent AZT] findings are an important step toward the goal of moving AIDS from "an inevitably fatal disease" to "a disease that can be controlled over time" through early treatment after infection.[9]

Dr. Samuel Broder, head of the National Cancer Institute and the man who claims the dubious credit for unleashing AZT upon the world, exposed in starker terms the impact of AIDS fatalism on treatment research:

> [The perception was that] treatments for AIDS would never be found: The cause was hopeless. [But] if you declare the patient terminal, you'll always be right.[10]

City and state health officials have also contributed to the deadly fatalism that assaults people with AIDS. For example, when the prestigious

New England Journal of Medicine published a study concluding that 15.2 percent of people diagnosed with AIDS in New York City had survived five or more years, that city's own health commissioner was quoted in the *New York Times* as being shocked; this 15.2 percent survival rate was, in his words, "greater than I would have intuitively expected it to be."[11] What the hell did that mean? Doesn't the health commissioner read, or believe, the data published by *his own department*? Shouldn't the health commissioner have known that *his own records* reflected a 15 percent survival rate? Shouldn't the *Times* reporter have asked whether he was guiding New York City's response to AIDS by a firm grasp of the data or by "intuition"?

In the same article, another AIDS expert explained the reasons for his surprise over the 15.2 percent survival rate: "People talk about AIDS as if it's an invariably fatal disease. . . ."[12] People? What people? Aren't doctors and AIDS experts the ultimate source of the fatalism? Is it enough for the health commissioner and other AIDS experts to just say, "Oops! Guess we were wrong about 100 percent mortality"?

With the possible exceptions of Congressmen Jesse Helms and William Dannemeyer, I don't believe that any government officials are actually gloating over the devastation brought about by AIDS. Still, it seems clear that the government and the medical establishment have permitted— indeed, are largely responsible for—the fatalism that blankets most discussions of the disease. The costs of this lie, measured in increased suffering and arguably in hastened deaths, have been staggering.

⊠ Rowdy AIDS activists and officials in charge of the government's AIDS response disagree about almost everything. Strangely, AIDS activists and government representatives have been united in their uncritical acceptance of the lie that AIDS = DEATH. How can one account for the fatalism promoted by representatives of AIDS-affected communities themselves?

As a survivor, I rail (to no avail) against the unfounded, glib, spirit-sucking assertion by some AIDS activists that the only cofactor that matters is time. While activists may reap short-term political gains from this assertion, it is disappointing that those who shout this seem unaware of—or unconcerned about—the impact this has on people with AIDS.

Once, after giving my "hope speech" during a public forum organized by the Gay Men's Health Crisis, I was angrily pulled aside by a gay man who worked in GMHC's Education Department. He begged me to stop saying that AIDS might not be 100 percent fatal. Shocked that a gay man would make such a request, I asked for reasons. He gave three: (1) efforts to persuade gay men to practice safer sex might be undermined because they would "take AIDS less seriously"; (2) it was bad for fund-raising; and (3) it would make lobbying for increased federal funding more difficult. "After all," he said, "if not everyone who gets it dies, then maybe AIDS isn't *really* the crisis we're being told it is."

I rejected his first and second points out of hand: "What?" I harrumphed. "Ninety percent mortality after three years isn't *good* enough? It has to be *100* percent mortality before people will practice safer sex and give money to AIDS service organizations?"

But the sad thing is that he was probably right to fear that right-wing congresspeople were looking for any excuse to justify not supporting increased funding for AIDS research. And it is historically true that the more strident that activists' demands became—the more dire the scenario presented—the more successful were lobbying efforts.

I asked this AIDS educator if he had considered what the consequences of the unfounded assertion that AIDS was invariably fatal might be for people *with* AIDS. He cold-bloodedly dismissed my concerns; as far as he was concerned, everybody with AIDS *is* going to die of it and our only hope was to get that message out to mainstream America, to motivate the country to demand a moon-launch approach to AIDS.

I participated in early strategy discussions among AIDS activists about how to "market" AIDS. As one of the first people with AIDS to testify in Congress, I was encouraged to present AIDS in the direst of terms and to emphasize the potential threat to heterosexuals. I strenuously objected to such a strategy because (a) there was no evidence that AIDS was spreading beyond the originally described risk groups, and (b) I thought that a strategy of scaring heterosexuals into believing the AIDS bogeyman was soon going to get them was dangerously shortsighted at a time when quarantining risk groups was considered, in some quarters, logistically feasible.

Activists argued that no one cared if "faggots" died and that scaring money out of the heterosexist Congress was our best hope. I clearly remember cringing when I heard the executive director of the Gay Men's Health Crisis compare AIDS to a "steaming locomotive roaring down the tracks" at the general, i.e., heterosexual, population. It wasn't true then, and data indicate that it's not true now; but it was a very successful political ploy.

Daily News reporter Heidi Evans is hopeful that AIDS activists will begin insisting that reporters acknowledge the phenomenon of *living* with AIDS in general, and the fact of long-term survival in specific. What gets covered and how it gets covered, she asserted, is definitely influenced by the activist agenda.

> Let's put it this way: That there *are* people who survive beyond a year or two or three is not well known. It's not well reported and it hasn't been one of those things that the AIDS advocacy community has pressed. I mean, you've been real busy talking about drugs, and a lot of progress has been made on those fronts. But the fact of long-term survival has not been a major idea that the activists have forced into the public's consciousness or into the consciousness of those of us who write about AIDS.

□ Whatever its source, the endless repetition of the lie that everyone dies from AIDS denies the reality of—but perhaps just as important, the possibility of—survival. Journalists, physicians, AIDS "experts," and activists must be extremely careful when they talk about AIDS. They must retain an awareness that how they speak about AIDS affects the way an individual *with* AIDS conceives her or his disease. And how an individual thinks about AIDS shapes the way he or she does battle with it.

NOTES

1. This editor's gratuitous, misinformed note preceded an excellent Associated Press article on long-term survival written by Paul Geitner, "Living with AIDS: Some Victims Live with It for Years," which ran, among other places, in the *Cedar Rapids Gazette,* Sunday, December 17, 1989, 20C.

2. Brand, David, "Surviving Is What I Do," reported by Scott Brown (Los Angeles) and Mary Cronin (New York), *Time* (May 2, 1988): 62–63.

3. I was interviewed by one of the authors of this article. She admitted that none of the reporters had thought to seek out AIDS survival statistics. I urged her to contact the CDC. I knew the article would prove disastrous when the reporter asked, "What's the CDC?" "The Centers for Disease Control," I answered. The silence at the other end betrayed no recognition. "In Atlanta. The government agency that keeps tracks of AIDS statistics." Did I have their number, she asked. Is it any wonder *Time*'s AIDS coverage has been so poor? I nevertheless gave the reporter the phone number for the CDC and informed her that there were *two* CDC studies on long-term survival trends, one of which had found 2.8 percent and one of which had found 15.2 percent. We had a discussion about what might account for the fact that two CDC researchers had reached dramatically different conclusions. There is no question that the reporter knew of both studies when she wrote the article; therefore, the failure to mention the more optimistic study can only have been deliberate.

4. AP wire story, untitled, September 15, 1989.

5. Lagnado, Lucette, "Dying AIDS Doc's Agony: Breaks Down in Tears During Courtroom Fight with City," *New York Post*, Sports Final, September 8, 1989.

6. It would obviously be easy for Health Department statisticians to include a column listing the numbers and percentages of those still *alive;* the fact that they don't is further evidence of the death bias that permeates official AIDS reports. This death bias, in turn, gets picked up and passed along uncritically by reporters.

7. Undated brochure entitled "Surgeon General's Report on Acquired Immune Deficiency Syndrome," printed by the U.S. Department of Health and Human Services and mailed to every U.S. household. According to the brochure, "This report was written personally by me to provide the necessary understanding of AIDS." "Me" refers to the well-meaning but—regarding survival probabilities—misinformed surgeon general, Dr. C. Everett Koop.

8. Often referred to by activists as the "AIDS Czar," Dr. Fauci's actual title is Director, National Institute of Allergy and Infectious Diseases, National Institutes of Health, and Coordinator, National Institutes of Health AIDS Program.

9. Dr. Anthony Fauci, quoted in Marlene Cimons, "AZT Found to Delay AIDS in Those Free of Symptoms," *Los Angeles Times*, August 18, 1989.

10. Dr. Samuel Broder, then chief of clinical trials at the National Cancer Institute, responding to expert explanations of why it took so long to begin to test AIDS drugs. Quoted in Randy Shilts, "AIDS/The Inside Story: The Epidemic's New Turning Point," *San Francisco Chronicle*, August 21, 1989.

11. New York City Health Commissioner Dr. Stephen Joseph, quoted in Gina Kolata, "15% of People with AIDS Survive 5 Years," *New York Times*, November 19, 1987.

12. Dr. Michael Grieco, quoted in Kolata.

"GUARANTEED TO DIE" OR YOUR MONEY BACK

The Price of Hope Denied

▨▨▨ For those of us residing in "the kingdom of the sick,"[1] it's hard to explain to those who are healthy that hope is like the air we breathe—it's that essential to survival. Shortly before he died, my friend and fellow long-term survivor, Max Navarre, eloquently articulated the impact that the myth of 100 percent mortality had on him:

> Does anyone consider the impact of [the] cult of the victim? Does anyone realize the power of the message "You are helpless. There is no hope for you"? I'm not immune to the reinforcement of hopelessness that surrounds me. That reinforcement causes despair, and I believe that despair kills people with AIDS as much as any of AIDS' physical manifestations. If we could truly believe in the possibility of *living* with AIDS, I think that survival figures would be higher.[2]

□ There are two kinds of hope: hope that expresses itself as a vague longing for a goal that may or may not be attainable, and hope empowered by the knowledge that the longed-for goal has been achieved by at least one person. The first requires blind faith; the other is more rational and based on probabilities.

A friend recently told me a story that illustrates the importance of both kinds of hope. For years, he said, athletes had been trying to run a mile in four minutes or less. But for the longest time, no one could crack the four-minute barrier.

Experts began to speculate that there must be inherent limitations in the human body that make this physical feat impossible. But all such expert opinion was proved wrong by one runner who, for the first time, ran a mile in under four minutes. (Perhaps he hadn't heard—or didn't believe—the experts' pessimism.)

Word of his achievement flashed around the world. Then, something even more amazing happened. Within a short time, others were suddenly able to run the mile in less than four minutes—including many who had tried before but failed.

Virtually every long-term survivor I know says that knowing another long-term survivor has been important in sustaining belief that he or she too might survive beyond predictions. I count myself very lucky that a month after I was diagnosed, I met Larry Goldstein. He was a handsome, vivacious gay man who owned a business and traveled the world despite the fact that he had developed KS in 1979 and had been retrospectively diagnosed with AIDS. When I met him in 1982, he was already a long-term survivor. Because the press rarely covered AIDS in the early years, Larry wasn't barraged by the relentless fatalism that today assaults anyone diagnosed with the disease.

I trace my belief in the possibility of my own survival to the example Larry unwittingly set for me at a crucial moment in my own conceptualization of AIDS. Larry radiated his belief that he was going to beat AIDS. In fact, he survived nine years![3]

⊠ Aside from the emotional toll that fatalism has taken on people with AIDS, the myth of 100 percent mortality has had a direct, negative impact on our physical well-being.

When first diagnosed with AIDS, many people examine their life-styles with the intention of identifying and removing behaviors that may be immunosuppressive. Perhaps those PWAs who give up sunbathing, marijuana, and alcohol should consider adding hopelessness to the list of immunosuppressants.

Western medicine only grudgingly acknowledges that hopelessness is immunosuppressive.[4] One of the most famous studies to demonstrate this involved rats that received electric shocks without any ability to control when or how often. Those that could shut off the shocks by pushing a lever remained comparatively immunocompetent.

Hopelessness also impinges on the health of PWAs through its impact on the physicians caring for us. A physician's belief that nothing can be done to alter the inexorable slide into death saps her or his will to aggressively diagnose, treat, and prophylax against the myriad diseases that, even with AIDS, are often treatable and preventable. "There is absolutely no question that proper patient management can contribute significantly to patient survival," said my own physician, Dr. Joseph Sonnabend.

> There's been an assumption on the part of some doctors . . . that there's nothing you can do. This is a terrible assumption that has cost lives. Of course, there are those who might say, "So what? If you're adding a few months or adding a year, what does it matter?" But I think it's very important that doctors not lose the sense of what we're doing, which is to maintain life *and* try to work out a cure for this disease.

The costs of cynicism and hopelessness were dramatically illustrated to me when I learned that one of the long-term survivors profiled in this book has recently become quite ill. I called to find out what was going on.

"It's MAI," he said. "I've had it for about nine months."

I asked him what medication he was taking for it. His reply shocked me.

"My doctor says MAI isn't treatable, so he hasn't prescribed anything."

I was flabbergasted! MAI is a *difficult* opportunistic infection to treat, but it is sometimes manageable—especially if diagnosed early and treated aggressively with a combination of anti-TB drugs. That any PWA should be allowed to go untreated for MAI is a sad comment on the corrosive impact of hopelessness and fatalism on physicians caring for people with AIDS.

Whether consciously or not, the federal government—and to a lesser extent, the medical establishment—has used the myth of 100 percent mortality to avoid full accountability for failing to quickly and aggressively pursue *treatment* research. After all, if everyone with AIDS is going to die anyway, why bother pursuing treatment at all? It is simply a historical fact that the government's pathetically inadequate AIDS response has focused primarily on prevention of HIV transmission and on vaccine development; people *with* AIDS have been largely abandoned as doomed.

⊠ What is so oppressive is the absolutism of the fatalism. It would be so easy for those who make authoritative pronouncements to leave open at least the theoretical *possibility* that some of us might survive. Such casual and careless fatalism—expressed with no apparent regard for the impact it might have on people with AIDS—hurts even more when found in pronouncements made by well-meaning friends intent on helping us "walk toward the light."

"I remember when a diagnosis was a death sentence," said Jim Graham, administrator of the Whitman Walker Clinic in Washington, a large gay/bisexual clinic that provides treatment and information to people affected by AIDS. "We didn't want to say that to people, and we didn't say it, but the unstated conclusion was that death was near."[5] Graham and other well-meaning care providers are being disingenuous: in nonverbal ways, they have communicated their "conclusion that death was near" loud and clear to anyone coming through their doors seeking care. Many PWAs dutifully proceed to fulfill the "unstated" expectations by giving up and dying on schedule.

Those of us who've insisted on the possibility of surviving have been patronized, handed Kübler-Ross, sent into therapy, or faced with the charge of having AIDS dementia.

One might think that news that a handful have survived would be enthusiastically received in those communities groaning under the burden of grief and suffering that AIDS leaves in its wake. But the reception afforded some long-term survivors has been far from supportive. One survivor I interviewed received death threats from the lover of someone who had died of the particular opportunistic disease that he had survived. Another was evicted from his apartment by a grief-stricken landlord whose lover had died of the disease that he continues to survive.

My own high profile as a long-term AIDS survivor has also led to some mean-spirited responses that reveal how deeply ingrained is the fatalism that surrounds AIDS. My first AIDS-defining opportunistic infection was cryptosporidiosis. Although cryptosporidium in an HIV-positive, immunocompromised individual was—and remains—on the list of infections that qualify one for a diagnosis of AIDS, some have suggested that because I didn't die, and because I wasn't initially diagnosed with KS or PCP, I shouldn't really count as a long-term survivor.[6]

It's interesting to examine their underlying message. If I had died from crypto in the summer of '82, no one would have questioned my "right" to an AIDS diagnosis. It is the fact that I *refused to die* that makes me suspect; and the fact of my survival apparently threatens some people's image of AIDS as invariably fatal.

There is a tautology built into the very definition of AIDS. When most people use that word, they mean the terminal stage of a spectrum of illness. But if you're only going to count as AIDS cases those that are terminal, then by definition the mortality rate will be 100 percent. Death from AIDS will become a self-fulfilling prophecy, and if you're not dead within three years, maybe you never really had AIDS in the first place. Such attitudes certainly send a powerful message to people struggling with AIDS that they'd better die on cue.

Something perverse in human nature seems to find extraordinary survival threatening. Robert Jay Lifton, author of *Death in Life,*[7] a book about survivors of Hiroshima, writes that:

> Survivors of various disasters have been targets of . . . hostility. In the London blitz, for instance, those who remained and thereby became survivors were frequently resented by those who fled the city. And the question asked of Jewish survivors of Nazi persecutions, "Why didn't you fight?" may unconsciously mean, "Why didn't you die?" (Survivors, of course, ask themselves the same question, either directly . . . or else indirectly when they ask of the dead, "Why didn't you live?" [The outsider] fears that his own life may have to be sacrificed in order to permit the now experienced survivor to continue his pattern of surviving others. He may unconsciously view the survivor as a kind of vampire who feeds on death, or even as part of a monstrous force which threatens to destroy the proper relationship between life and death.

☐ Will we ever be able to measure the damage done by the media's refusal to seek out long-term survivors? How many PWAs have obediently fulfilled the gloom-and-doom prophecy?

Believing that AIDS is universally fatal, our physicians, friends, family, and lovers humor our illusions and ration out their emotional strength, certain that, however draining, however horrible it may be to watch the progress of AIDS, at least the *end* is inevitable. Admitting the possibility of survival means that people around us may have to suffer the disappointment of our hopes along with us in a new way. If death from AIDS is *not* inevitable, then each death is uniquely painful. And each struggle to survive is uniquely empowering.

NOTES

1. Sontag, Susan. *Illness as Metaphor* (New York: Farrar, Straus & Giroux, 1977), p. 3.

2. Navarre, Max, "Fighting the Victim Label," *October Magazine*, Issue #43, Winter 1987, 143.

3. Although I lost touch with him, I learned through friends that Larry Goldstein died in 1988. But none of them knew whether he died of AIDS. For all I know, he was hit by a cab! New York City has always been potentially lethal.

4. See, for example, what psychoneuroimmunologist George Solomon refers to as "the literature on helplessness-hopelessness":

Laudenslager, M.D., et al., "Coping and immunosuppression: Inescapable but not escapable shock suppresses lymphocyte proliferation," *Science*, 221 (1983): 568–580; Levy, S.M., "Behavior as biologic response modifier: The psychoimmunoendocrine network and tumor immunology," *Behavioral Medicine Abstracts*, 6 (1985): 1–4; and Schmale, A.H., et al., "The affect of hopelessness and the development of cancer," *Psychosomatic Medicine*, 28 (1966): 714–721.

5. Hilts, Philip J., "Major Changes for Health System Seen in Wake of the AIDS Finding," *New York Times*, August 19, 1989.

6. I had to go so far as to *publish* my biopsy results along with a note from my physician affirming that I do in fact have AIDS in order to silence those who were circulating the rumor that I was only *posing* as a person with AIDS. See Callen, Michael, "Are You Now or Have You Ever Been," *PWA Coalition Newsline*, Issue 40, January 1989, 34–37.

7. Lifton, Robert Jay. *Death in Life: Survivors of Hiroshima*. New York: Basic Books, 1982. Thanks to Victor Zonana for bringing this book to my attention.

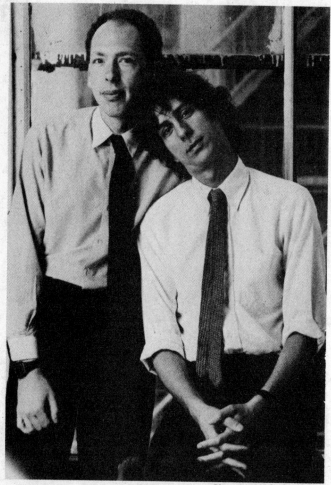

Michael Callen, right, and his lover, Richard Dworkin.

LUCK, CLASSIC COKE, AND THE LOVE OF A GOOD MAN

▨▨▨ One of the most important recommendations contained in the Denver Principles—the founding manifesto of the PWA self-empowerment movement—is this:

> People with AIDS must be included in all AIDS forums with equal credibility as other participants, to share their own experiences and knowledge.[1]

As PWA activist Bobbi Campbell, a coauthor of the Denver Principles, put it, people with AIDS are the *real* experts.

What I had learned about long-term AIDS survival from talking to statisticians, physicians, and other experts was interesting, but I wasn't satisfied. I decided to interview those whom I considered to be, finally, the real experts: other long-term survivors.

But before I could do that, I realized that I'd have to examine my own case, if only to identify the kinds of questions I would ask other survivors.

▨ In the last few years, I've been asked dozens of times why I think I've survived. I usually quip, "Luck, Classic Coke, and the love of a good man." I'm only half-joking.

Whenever I seriously contemplate why I have survived AIDS for eight years, I keep coming back to one word: luck. The plain fact is that I *have* been lucky. Like my AIDS activism, my experience of AIDS has been eccentric and idiosyncratic.

Even at my sickest, I've never been all that sick. Although I might have died from cryptosporidiosis, my first opportunistic infection, I didn't. No one quite knows why. I had crypto because my immune system was seriously depressed, but I apparently had just enough immune response left to force a recovery. Since the summer of 1982, the diarrhea and weight loss have come and gone, but they've been manageable.

The bacterial pneumonias that I seem to get every winter are the most frightening and annoying complication of AIDS I've endured. Every time a PWA gets short of breath, everyone jumps to the conclusion that it's PCP. Although I've been on medication to prevent PCP since 1982, a small percentage of PWAs receiving PCP prophylaxis occasionally develop PCP anyway. So I always have to go through a week of terror, endure X rays and blood gas tests, and live with the threat of another bronchoscopy hanging over my head. Fortunately, it has always turned out not to be PCP, and the bacterial pneumonias have always responded to antibiotics.

I have been hospitalized with shingles and I've received several blood transfusions, but not for anemia. They were given, instead, to correct an immune-complex problem.

I have Kaposi's sarcoma, but again, I've been lucky. I only have about a dozen lesions, and they are small and slow-growing.[2] Except for two tiny spots on my face, the lesions are in places usually covered by clothes, which permits me to lead a relatively normal life; I've been spared the embarrassment of strangers staring in horror at my disfigurement.

I had a major lymphoma scare in early 1989, but after three endoscopies that yielded "suggestive but inconclusive" biopsies, the best-guess diagnosis is that I have a bizarre, "lymphoma-like" B-cell proliferation lining my esophagus and small intestine.

Having AIDS has felt very much like the serious, chronic mononucleosis I had in high school. Fevers, fatigue, and swollen lymph glands are like old friends; we've been through so much together.

I have never had more than 200 T-helper cells since first being tested in 1981, and cytomegalovirus (CMV)—a herpes virus—can regularly be cultured from my semen, urine, and blood. And though I consider it meaningless, I am an HIV *factory;* I apparently have high levels of HIV viral activity, which makes it easy for researchers to culture HIV from my blood. Being such a well-known HIV heretic, I find it amusingly ironic that one New York lab uses HIV isolated from my blood to make antibody testing materials.

☒ I'm certain that one reason why I'm alive today is because I've managed to avoid PCP—the pneumonia that has killed most of those who have died from AIDS. Once again, my doctor, Joe Sonnabend, deserves the credit for his foresight.

The reason I've never had PCP is that he insisted—well ahead of his time and despite the contempt of his colleagues—that his patients take two double-strength Bactrim tablets daily to prevent PCP. That wasn't luck; that was just good doctoring.

Actually, I often feel that I'm alive today more because of what I *didn't* do than because of what I did do.

Like most PWAs, in the early days following my diagnosis I was desperate to *do* something—to take some drug, *any* drug. But Dr. Sonnabend always counseled caution. While many of the new friends I had met in PWA support groups were flying to France for HPA-23, smuggling Ribavirin in from Mexico, or seeking some mysterious "cure" in Barbados, I reluctantly took nothing but Bactrim. As I watched many friends, who in desperation had grasped at the latest drug *du jour,* end up suffering and dying as much from drug-related toxicities as from AIDS itself, I began to see the wisdom of Dr. Sonnabend's advice.

Instead of bone-marrow transplants, high-dose interferon, full-body radiation, combination chemotherapy, and ever more toxic nucleoside analogues such as AZT and ddI, I have explored comparatively benign therapies such as plasmapheresis,[3] low-dose naltrexone,[4] egg lipids,[5] high-dose acyclovir,[6] and Itraconazole.[7]

My doctor's philosophy regarding AIDS treatments is simple and has stood me in good stead: In the absence of proven therapies, concentrate on interventions that may or may not help but that you are reasonably certain won't harm you. Although most of my fellow AIDS activists seem unable to comprehend it, no treatment is better than the wrong treatment. Not believing that I'll likely be dead tomorrow if I don't do something drastic, I've had the luxury of waiting and watching. I figure if a drug ever comes along that *cures* AIDS, I'll hear about it in plenty of time to benefit.

▨ In my survival trilogy, Coca-Cola is meant as a metaphor for simple pleasures. Whenever I'm feeling low and looking for a reason to keep struggling, I remind myself that sugar is a sufficient reason to live.

Macro/veggie types cringe every time I jokingly credit Classic Coke for having contributed to my survival, but the truth is, I drink scandalous amounts of it. (My goal as a cook is to someday prepare a meal that brings me more pleasure than the cola that I wash it down with.)

▨ Might my survival have something to do with genetics?

Somewhat immodestly, my mom thinks so. When I melodramatically phoned my parents in 1982 to tell them that I had a fatal disease and would probably be dead within six months, my mom was having none of it. "You're made from good American Indian and Pennsylvania Dutch stock," she said, meaning that obviously I'd therefore lick whatever this problem was.

In any case, I'm certain that I would have died long ago if I hadn't enjoyed the love and support of family, friends, and my lover. And I'm metaphysical enough to admit that this love and support have seen me through the dark times, when it was tempting to just give up.

My family has been as supportive as it's been possible to be living eight hundred and fifty miles away. Regular phone calls to check up on me, and unsolicited offers of financial and practical assistance, have left no doubt that I am loved, despite our past painful battles over my gayness and my atheism.

My high profile in the national media is very hard on them, but my parents say they are proud of my AIDS activism. They tell me that they realize that my speaking out against the many injustices committed against people with AIDS is consistent with the lessons they taught me as a child; but I'm aware that they have paid a price for my visibility. My mother is a schoolteacher and she can always tell when I've appeared on national television, because people treat her differently the next day. Some are solicitous; others stare and move away.

⊠ Knowing other PWAs has also played an important role in my survival. I have found networking with others similarly situated to be invaluable. And though it's been painful to lose so many comrades, the emotional support provided by PWA support groups has been very sustaining.

But it is to my lover that I feel I owe my life. There is no question in my mind that I would not be alive today if, at a crucial moment in the process of coming to terms with AIDS, I hadn't met my lover, Richard Dworkin. I consider myself unspeakably lucky to have met him when I did.

The worst part about being diagnosed wasn't the thought of dying. It was believing that I would die without ever having known the love of another man. I'd had lots of sex, but I'd never really had a lover—as in living with someone and wanting to grow old and grumpy with him. And so when the AIDS sentence was pronounced, I felt like factory seconds—damaged merchandise. It never occurred to me that anyone would risk loving me now that I had AIDS.

Shortly before I was officially diagnosed with AIDS, I had decided to finally get serious about pursuing my music. I placed an ad looking for lesbian and gay musicians.

When Richard arrived for his audition, I explained that I had GRID. I wanted to lay that on the table in case he was freaked out about it, or in case he didn't want to invest time in a group knowing that the lead singer had a life expectancy shorter than that of a garage band. To make a long story short, I got a drummer *and* a lover out of that audition.

At the lowest moment of my life, when my guard was down, he . . . pounced. I couldn't have been more shocked, and I in fact pushed him away. I said: "You don't understand. I have GRID!"

He said something like "I understand, but I think we're meant for each other." I asked him why he would risk getting involved with somebody with a fatal illness that was probably contagious.

His answer amazed me. "I'm a gay man living in New York City," he said. "I'm going to have to deal with this disease sooner or later. I may as well begin now."

I had no snappy comeback; I was dumbfounded. I asked him whether he was worried that he might get this horrible disease from me. He said two things: (1) He was no stranger to promiscuity himself and if he ever came down with GRID, he certainly wouldn't assume he got it from me; and (2) he too had been reading about this mysterious new disease and had independently concluded that only those people who had abused their immune systems over a long period of time were getting it. Since his history of sexually transmitted diseases was minimal, he didn't think he was at very great risk for AIDS.

Eight years later, it still amazes me that he was crazy enough to take a chance on loving someone who everybody thought would be dead within six months.

Richard hates when I say that he's the key to my survival because it implies that if he were to leave me, I'd die. Or that if I die, he must not have loved me enough. I know my illness has been a burden to him—one that he has, by and large, borne without complaint. Like most relationships, ours is complex. I would probably be hard to live with *without* the added complication of AIDS. Like other people, we have our fights and our incompatibilities. But each of us realized long ago that, for better or worse, we'll love each other for as long as we live.

Richard has a complex reaction to my involvement in AIDS politics. Because I speak frequently to the media, I'm constantly being asked to talk about our relationship. (Journalists seem to have a fascination with why a person would be crazy enough to fall in love with someone with AIDS.) He's essentially shy and private and doesn't like it when I talk about him in public. And yet, he has always encouraged my political activities. He helps shape my thinking, edits my writing, and nurses my wounds when I return from battle.

His biggest complaint about my AIDS activism, aside from its impact on my health, is that it has prevented me from pursuing singing and songwriting. It's only thanks to him that I finally released *Purple Heart,* my first album.[8] He produced it and played drums on it. But I barely remember recording *Purple Heart,* because I was distracted and preoccupied by my PWA activism. I finished the album the same week that *Surviving and Thriving with AIDS,* volume 2, went to the printer. I felt like I had given birth to twins, and that the labor had been particularly protracted. What should have been a joyful achievement—the release of my first album—was compromised by sheer physical exhaustion from having too many balls in the air at one time. Whatever credit is deserved for *Purple Heart* really belongs to Richard for having done the thankless grunt work that made it possible, and for having pushed me to do it in the first place.

Can an atheist get away with saying that he feels incredibly blessed?

▨ My friends have their own theories about why I've survived. Some say it's because I have a sense of purpose—a reason to live—and that I'm passionately committed to life. They point to my political activism as Exhibit A.

But I've often wondered if they're right. The problem is, my AIDS activism has been a double-edged sword. It has given me a reason to live, but it has also nearly killed me. On the one hand, feeling the first warning signs of yet another bout of bacterial pneumonia, I've said to myself, "I can't die yet; I have congressional testimony to give!" On the other hand, my schedule would probably kill a *healthy* person!

The frenetic pace of my life has meant that I've been able to rationalize to myself that I mustn't be all *that* sick because if I was, I couldn't keep so busy; but the sheer, physical wear and tear on my body, combined with the viciousness of political battles, makes me wonder whether my activism has been good or bad for my health.[9]

▨ Having examined my own survival, I had a sense of what questions I would ask other survivors. Would they be like me? Were there patterns? I was eager to talk to the *real* experts.

NOTES

1. "The Denver Principles: Statement from the Advisory Committee of People with AIDS" was first formulated at a historic AIDS conference held in Denver in 1983. The entire manifesto is reprinted in *Surviving and Thriving with AIDS: Collected Wisdom*, volume 2, Michael Callen, ed., New York: PWA Coalition, Inc., 1988, 294–295.

2. It is one of the most glaring examples of how poor the scientific response to AIDS has been that the relationship between Kaposi's sarcoma and AIDS remains mysterious after more than a decade since AIDS was first described. No one has satisfactorily explained why KS appears to be an AIDS-related complication for gay and bisexual men but not (with rare exceptions) for members of other "risk groups." No one knows why in some people it is rapidly progressive while in others it is indolent and non-life-threatening. Dr. Robert Gallo's lab announced with great fanfare in 1988 that it had isolated a KS growth factor in the blood of PWAs. Those of us with KS have waited in vain for a follow-up report on what that might mean

for us clinically, but so far, no new information of any practical value has been forthcoming.

3. Plasmapheresis is a blood-cleansing process during which one's blood is removed a pint at a time and then centrifuged to separate the blood cells from the plasma. The plasma is then thrown away and the blood cells get returned to you, along with fluid to replace the volume of plasma that has been removed. This cumbersome, labor-intensive process removes interferon, tumor necrosis factor, and miscellaneous viral debris from the blood. Dr. Sonnabend believes the delay in my developing KS after my initial opportunistic infection may be attributable, in part, to the fact that I have been plasmapheresed.

4. Naltrexone is an opiate-blocker usually prescribed to prevent heroin addicts from getting high. As a potential therapy for AIDS, one 50 mg. pill is dissolved in icky-tasting cherry syrup that is taken in virtually homeopathic doses to reduce the levels of circulating interferon, which are usually elevated in PWAs. A detailed report of a promising study of naltrexone in PWAs has been submitted for publication to a major medical journal. Those interested in reading a preliminary report should consult the following abstract: Bernard Bihari, et al., "Low Dose Naltrexone in the Treatment of AIDS: Long Term Follow-Up Results," Fifth International AIDS Conference, 1989, Book of Abstracts, M.C.P.62, 552.

5. Egg lipids, also known as AL-721, are vile, sebaceous substances that look like and are about as appetizing as earwax. Several years ago, prominent AIDS researcher Dr. Robert Gallo wrote a letter, which was published in a major medical journal, in which he described AL-721 as effective in preventing HIV from infecting uninfected cells. He regarded it as one of the most promising therapies in need of testing. The main advantage of lipids is that they are apparently nontoxic, since they are basically a food rather than a drug. The little research that has been done hasn't demonstrated any dramatic efficacy and I stopped taking lipids due to their dubious worth and the terrible inconvenience of traveling with them.

6. Acyclovir, also known as Zovirax, is an antiherpes drug that probably controls cytomegalovirus, Epstein-Barr virus, and the other herpes virus activity that plagues people with AIDS. Preliminary evidence suggests that taken in high doses, it is effective at preventing CMV retinitis and other common complications of CMV infection in people with AIDS. Although like AZT it is a nucleoside analogue, it works through a different mechanism of action and has none of AZT's fabled toxicity.

7. Itraconazole is an antifungal medication manufactured by Jansen Pharmaceuticals and imported by the PWA Health Group from Mexico. I take it to prevent candida and cryptococcal meningitis.

8. Those interested can order *Purple Heart* by sending a $10 check or money order payable to Significant Other Records to P.O. Box 1545, Canal Street Station, New York, New York 10013. Please specify album or cassette.

9. I'm told that technically speaking, Kaposi's sarcoma isn't really a sarcoma; one cancer expert said I should think of a KS lesion as a bruise that doesn't heal. I have a strange image that I can't shake. My first KS lesions appeared during an unusually ugly political battle; I have come to associate each new lesion with a particular political ambush.

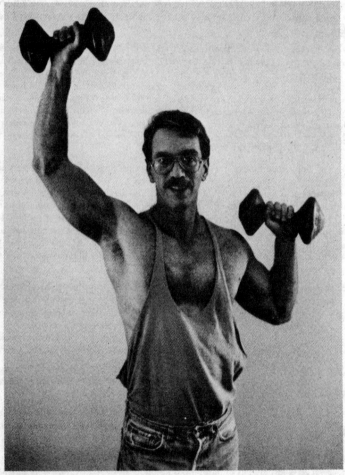

The Reverend Steven Pieters.

Photo © 1989 by Lawrence T. Root.

THE REVEREND STEVEN PIETERS

"Believe in the possibility."

▨▨▨ I had flown out to Los Angeles to sing at the 1987 Los Angeles AIDS Walkathon. I could hardly believe my ears when, during the ceremony, the handsome, body-built opening speaker identified himself as Steve Pieters, a thirty-year-old gay man who had just celebrated his third anniversary as a person with AIDS. When the ceremony ended, I dashed over to meet him. He quickly agreed to be interviewed for this book.

Steve's cozy, lived-in living room was piled with books and papers. Like many PWA activists, he spends a great deal of his time writing about living with AIDS, and during our interview, his computer's printer buzzed in the background. He and his cats ushered me to a comfortable couch located next to a bookshelf full of videos of musicals and comedies.

I was nervous. Steve was my first interview and I wanted to ask all the right questions in a way that wasn't offensive or prying. Steve quickly put me at ease and suggested we start with his personal AIDS history.

Looking back on his life prior to diagnosis, Steve felt that the warning signs of AIDS had been there all along. "My immune system was worn down by stress, the stress of my job, the stress of a failed love relationship and too many binge drugs," he explained. "I had my weekends where I partied too hard." He recalled that beginning in 1982, he suffered health problems that he now believes presaged AIDS: bouts of viral illnesses, such as hepatitis and cytomegalovirus; thrush; and a mysterious foot fungus.

He wasn't diagnosed with full-blown AIDS until April 1984, when he developed both Kaposi's sarcoma and systemic, B-cell lymphoma. "I was pretty healthy for about the next year, although one health care professional told me I wouldn't see 1985."

I decided to start with the million-dollar question: Why did he think he was still alive more than three years after his diagnosis?

"I think that I'm healthy because I've pulled together all the resources that I can to survive, plus luck, or God's grace—depending on your point of view."

I squirmed; not being at all religious, it had never occurred to me that I would encounter a gay man who would credit God with his survival. "Which do you think," I asked. "Luck or God's grace?"

"God's grace," he smiled. "You see, I'm a minister with the Metropolitan Community Church." My eyes widened as I tried in vain to conceal my horror. Steve had clearly encountered many gay atheists like me and was more than willing to explain his faith.

"I believe that's God's grace has permitted me to survive. But," he added quickly, "I'm sometimes uncomfortable saying that. Because what does that mean about people who've *not* survived? That God's grace wasn't there? No, I don't think so. I have certainly seen that other people who've died have experienced God's grace."

I asked him what he thought was the difference between luck and God's grace.

"Well, grace to me is more intentional—like, God picked somebody out and said, 'This person will be graced.' Whereas luck is more . . . arbitrary."

Not wanting to be rude and express my profound disgust with religion, I decided to switch subjects. I asked Steve if he gave any credit to Western medicine.

"Well, in 1985, I started on Suramin," he explained. I had heard about the Suramin trials. They were notorious in AIDS activist circles because so many people with AIDS died because the NIH took so long to alert participants and physicians to the serious side effects of the drug. "I was one of the first to take Suramin," he recalled proudly. "And within six weeks, my KS lesions had disappeared. They did biopsies and they came back negative. Also, before Suramin, I had been in fourth-stage lymphoma, but now the tests showed I had no lymphoma left. Everything was in complete remission."

But the side effects of Suramin nearly killed him.

"I felt like I was on the bottom of a bowl of Jell-O. Strangely, I never had the fevers or other things that other guys on Suramin did. I took Suramin for thirty-nine weeks, which is twelve weeks longer than the next longest person was on it. I started wasting away in late September of 1985. By the end of October, I was sleeping about eighteen hours a day, and anytime I'd stand up, I would black out. I was really sick. They kept saying, 'We don't know what's going on. The cancer's not there; nothing's happening.' The National Institutes of Health finally advised my doctors to check my adrenal glands and, sure enough, there was Addison's disease—adrenal insufficiency.

"I came very close to death the night they discovered the problem with my adrenal glands. My blood pressure was down to 50 over 30. I had a near-death experience at that point. I was beginning to suffer neurologic side effects. The nerves became so inflamed that I couldn't see. The left side of my body atrophied. The muscles just all wasted away and I was sleeping most of the time. I couldn't hold a glass. I couldn't make things work. Everything was going. Coming up on my second anniversary of diagnosis, I was pretty sure I was dying."

It was hard to imagine the narrator of this tale, bursting with health and vigor, as someone wasting away and near death. Fortunately, Steve stopped the drug in the nick of time and recovered entirely from Suramin's debilitating side effects.

"I remember I got terribly constipated toward the end of February '86. Suddenly, when that cleared, I started getting better, and I haven't had any major health problems since that. My cancer is in complete remission and I've not had any further opportunistic infections. My blood counts are within normal ranges, and I'm doing very well.

"I don't think it was any coincidence that my cancers went into complete remission on Suramin. I think that Suramin gave me the push that I needed to go into remission, even though it didn't work for anybody else. However, I think that I created the conditions for healing before I started on Suramin."

He then launched into a passionate encomium about his doctor—a theme that resonated comfortably with my own experience.

"I *love* my doctor. She's absolutely wonderful. Her name's Alexandra Levine. She is the only doctor in my experience who does not preclude the search for alternative treatments and therapies. She's very open to working together with the patient in creating wellness—creating the conditions for healing. *And* she's a topflight scientist."

I asked him if she was the person who had told him he wouldn't live to see 1985.

"Oh, no. It was a nurse who said that. As I recall, I did not confront her. I just sort of took in what she said. My own doctors have *never* given me a prognosis. Dr. Levine has *never* told me how long I have. She doesn't believe in that sort of thing. Dr. Levine has a monthly update for the people with AIDS in her studies. There were probably thirty of us in the room and the subject came up about my health and wellness, and there was a reaction to her announcement that I was in complete remission. She was asked, 'Why isn't anybody studying the people who are well?' And her response was, 'Well, we're too busy studying lots of other things.' And then I said, 'Well, I've heard that there are over one hundred people around the country who have been diagnosed for three years or more.' And she said, 'Oh, there's got to be more than that! There are three or four of them in this room.' And she asked us to raise our hands, and there were four people out of thirty who had survived AIDS for three years or more.

"Before I was diagnosed," Steve explained, "I didn't believe survival was possible. I had no concrete reason to believe it when I was diagnosed. There wasn't a lot of publicity about long-term survivors in 1984. But I was reading a lot of books like *Getting Well Again* and *The Relaxation Response*, books that talked about how doctors don't know everything. And particularly about AIDS, doctors don't know everything and the chances are that there are going to be people who are going to survive! And so, I thought, why not *me?*

"Actually, when I was in my pre-AIDS state I was scared to death. I was paralyzed by my fear and I wouldn't go out of the house. I found it difficult to even go to the grocery store because there were people there. But as soon as I was diagnosed I started articulating that I was going to follow a plan of living with AIDS, rather than dying.

"At the time, I was not aware of the PWA self-empowerment movement. Actually," he recalled, "I got the idea of *living* with AIDS from a social worker at AIDS Project Los Angeles (APLA), and I also got it from my faith. Mine is a God of love, not a God of death. And so I believe that God wants us to be healthy. I believe that God is greater than AIDS. I used to be really, really scared of death. But now I believe that facing death, facing my mortality, the reality that I *will* die one day, really helped me focus on life. Especially after the near-death experience. There is value in embracing the fact that we all will die, and accepting that as a reality of life. It has somehow freed me to live more fully.

I was fascinated by his mention of a near-death experience. I asked him to describe it.

"Well, I didn't fall into a tunnel and see a white light at the end with familiar faces or anything like that," he laughed. "I could feel less and less of my body. My awareness, my consciousness was retreating. The doctors were working away on me; my blood pressure was really low. The specific moment that I remember was when they were trying to get blood from my arm and they were not able to get it and they said 'Squeeze your hand, Steve' and my hand didn't move and I remember just closing my eyes. I had practiced praying with each breath. And so I prayed as I breathed and that really helped. It allowed me to remove myself from that situation and relax and concentrate on my breathing.

"As I did that, I suddenly found myself floating above the scene and feeling real peace, a sense that none of this bullshit matters, a sense of total unity with the best feelings I'd ever had, the best orgasm I'd ever had. It was an ecstatic experience, and yet, grounded in peacefulness.

"I didn't really remember it at first. It took me a few days for it to come back. But when it did, I knew I had lost my fear of death. I'm just not scared of it."

He kept returning to the subject of religion. It was clear that he was very sincere in his faith and that he had taken great comfort from his religious beliefs. Perhaps sensing less resistance on my part, he again attempted to explain the role that he felt God had played in his survival.

"When I refer to 'God' and 'God's grace,' I am referring to the mystery of God. I don't pretend to understand it. For example, in the book of Job, when they talk about why the righteous have to suffer and the answer comes in a voice of the wind and it says: 'Where were you when God created the universe?' And to me, that's *an* answer. I mean, where *was* I when God created the universe?"

I couldn't resist: "At the baths?"

He laughed good-naturedly and I decided I should again quickly change the subject. I asked Steve if he had been politically active before his AIDS diagnosis.

"Well," he explained, "as pastor of Metropolitan Community Church of Hartford, I was a local gay activist and did a lot of media projects around gay activism. I have always enjoyed writing too. So when I was diagnosed, I started writing about my experiences. And I got involved with AIDS Project Los Angeles in April of '85. Back then I was *the* media person. I had no problem being public. Right from the beginning they pushed me in front of cameras and said, 'This is a person with AIDS who can articulate his experiences.' And shortly after that they put me on their board of directors. Political activism has been part of my survival strategy. Getting outside of myself. Doing volunteer work around AIDS as much as I could."

Steve seemed to enjoy being a highly visible long-term survivor. I asked him what reactions he had encountered.

He smiled. "People often want to touch me and to know what I've done. It's always, 'What did you *do* to heal yourself?' "

"What do you tell them?" I asked.

"Believe in the possibility, first of all," he advised. "That's real important."

"But what advice do you give about diet and treatments and things like that?" I asked.

"For the past decade, I've been into bodybuilding and nutrition. So I have continued to exercise when I've been physically able and I have really tried to keep up on vitamins and fresh vegetables and fruit and cut down or out on alcohol and tobacco. I haven't completely eliminated red meat, but I have eliminated tobacco. I haven't completely eliminated caffeine, but I've cut down.

"I got turned off to macrobiotics early in my diagnosis, because I saw somebody who was doing it and he was wasting away and getting weaker and weaker and the macrobiotics were not helping him, at least as far as I could see. And I've seen a couple of other people go that route and not do well on it. So I never was attracted to macrobiotics. I like to do what I call common-sense nutrition.

"I've also done a lot of alternative therapies, although I haven't done everything," he said. "And I'm *definitely* not a fan of Louise Hay!"

I asked him why he was so vehemently opposed to someone who had so many PWA followers. He explained that he'd had several run-ins with what he referred to as "Louise Hay fanatics."

"One time I was on my way out the door to go to Burger King and a Louise Hay fan asked me where I was going. And I said, 'To Burger King.' And he said, 'You want to kill yourself?' And I said, 'Well, no. I believe in not depriving myself of things that I like.' And you know what? He's dead and I'm alive.

"I've been to Louise Hay's group sometimes and she does have great group energy and a lot of people get a lot out of it, but I tell you the people who start failing feel guilty. And that's not good."

I asked him if he had ever done the AIDS Mastery—a workshop intended to help people cope with AIDS.

"I have not done things like that," Steve said. "Their attitude is, 'I'm going to teach you how to survive AIDS, dear.' Well, thank you, but I've lived with it for five years. I think I've done it myself; I've discovered my own way. I'm sure that they're doing a lot of good work and a lot of people are very enthusiastic about them, but I've found my own path.

"I go to a therapist who works in conjunction with a body worker who is a psychic healer. I lie on the table and she puts her hands over me and removes the toxins and things, and brings up things that I have to deal with in therapy. And I don't know how it works, but I believe in it. I have every reason to believe that it's been central to my survival. I did acupuncture when I was first diagnosed, and stress reduction as well, to stop smoking cigarettes.

"I still smoke marijuana, although I have cut down considerably. People look askance at me because they say it's not good for my immune system, but it increased my appetite when I needed to eat and it calmed my nausea."

"I have done lots of laughter therapy, like Norman Cousins recommends. I bought a VCR and have lots of sitcoms on tapes and musical comedy. I try to keep myself entertained and try to keep in touch with the child within me."

I wanted to try to pin him down about drugs. I asked him if he was on any medications. He startled me by indicating that he was not on any form of PCP prevention.

"I've chosen not to do PCP prophylaxis or to take AZT," he said. "I feel I did my time on experimental drugs and I'm doing fine without it. Why tamper with success?"

I mentioned that the medical literature on long-term survival with other so-called terminal diseases suggests that having goals is another survival characteristic. I asked him if he had any goals.

"Through the period when I was on Suramin—when I was the sickest—I really didn't have a goal," he admitted. "But then again, I felt like I wasn't quite done with life yet. Now, I want to write a book. I think I'll call it *Tap Dancing Through AIDS,*" he laughed. "It'll be about coping and surviving."

Any other goals, I asked?

"I want to participate on a wider level in the AIDS movement."

Thinking of my own complicated reaction to my AIDS activism, I asked him if he didn't sometimes resent the price that being publicly identified as a person with AIDS—and especially as a long-term survivor—can extract. His answer surprised me.

"I get a lot of resentment from people who have lost lovers, from people who are doing poorly. In fact, I had a death threat from the lover of someone who had died. The surviving lover was very angry; he felt that I hadn't visited his lover in the hospital enough, and when it got out that I had gone into complete remission, he called me up and threatened my life. I changed my number to an unlisted one."

And I thought *I'd* had it rough. At least those who were threatened by my long-term survival hadn't resorted to death threats.

"I've also had people pushing diets and fads try to get me to endorse their product, since I am a well person with AIDS. I refuse to do that."

We shared horror stories, and it was oddly healing for me to know that at least one other long-term survivor had encountered surprising hostility and exploitation. I mentioned my bizarre encounter with a gay man who ordered me to stop talking about survival because it was bad for fund-raising.

"I had the same experience!" he said. "It was *amazing!* I was on the board of AIDS Project Los Angeles when I went into remission. I started telling people there about my good news, and the person in charge of fund-raising said to me, 'Please don't tell anybody about that because it'll be real bad for fund-raising if it gets out that people are doing well.'

"My reaction was, 'No, people need to hear that.' Actually, I was really pissed. I feel it's my *duty* is to spread hope. To let people know that there are people who are living long past the designated time 'allotted.' I've been traveling extensively and do a great deal of public speaking. The fact is that I'm *thriving*. I'm surviving. I'm well. And people love to hear that, and they need to hear it, because there's so little hope out there."

I wanted to know what support system he had to help him cope with all the pressure.

"I've been sick for five years," he explained matter-of-factly. "And family and friends just can't keep up with that. My family has been very supportive from a distance, but they can't take actually being here. When I was first sick here in Los Angeles, it was my experience that gay men in Los Angeles stayed away from me in droves. And it was my lesbian friends who really took care of me. Specifically, there was a radical black lesbian feminist who, when I was quite sick, was the one person I could count on seeing. She brought me groceries, she sat with me and we watched TV. She was right there for me.

"The last time that I was sick, there were a couple of men who would come over and visit and bring me groceries and do things for me, but they wouldn't sit and be with me. I've been very lonely for gay men through-out this—for intimacy. And I don't mean sex, necessarily, although that's nice too. But to just be held and cuddled."

"What *about* your love life?" I pried.

He laughed. "I don't have a lover. I did briefly in the second year of my diagnosis. Not having a lover is something that I've really grieved for, and I continue to grieve," he said pensively.

"Well," I charged ahead shamelessly, "then what about your sex life?"

"I went through a period where I was impotent," he explained. "The Suramin destroyed my testosterone. And so, for a while, it just wasn't an issue. But since I've been off Suramin and they started giving me testoster-one every three weeks, I get a testosterone rush about three days after I get the shot and it carries me through, and so occasionally I have safe sex. I will go months at a time without it.

"I don't need sex as much as I used to. I don't want a hassle. I mean, if I had a lover it would be one thing, but I'm just not into going out and picking up strangers anymore and having to explain to them safer sex and my health situation. It's difficult. I've been rejected a lot."

We talked for a while about the good ol' days of pre-AIDS sexuality. We lamented the long-lost innocence and waxed sloppily nostalgic.

"I enjoyed promiscuity a lot as I was going through it," Steve explained. "I enjoyed that freedom and I felt it was a celebration of our sexuality and of who we are. I had grown up feeling ashamed of my sexuality. I really hated myself for being gay until I was about twenty-three. And then when I came out in 1975 and decided that that shame was foolish, it was just such a liberating experience, because I suddenly was able to meet men. I thoroughly enjoyed the gay life-style of the seventies. I wouldn't change it for anything. I think that if I had stayed in the closet and not experienced that, I would have suffocated or committed suicide."

I could chat about sex for hours, but since Steve had told me that he had to be somewhere soon, I reluctantly abandoned my favorite topic and moved on to other issues. I asked him if he had found being in support groups with other PWAs to be helpful.

"When I was first diagnosed, joining a support group really helped," he said. "It demystified AIDS. It made me feel like I wasn't some sort of freak. It was a very healing process for me to meet other PWAs and to get integrated into the community. And it was there that I learned about treatments and things. But once I got past about two years in the support groups I went through a terrible depression because everybody had died that had been diagnosed when I was. I just got tired of all the death, so I pulled back and eliminated my involvement with support groups. Now, I'd like to see support groups for people who've been diagnosed for a couple of years. I really think there are very different issues which have to be dealt with."

As our interview was ending, I asked him if he had any final comments. He thought for a moment and then said, "I believe that one of the alternative therapies for me—and this may sound strange—has been being gay! Let's just say that I believe in fairies, and I always have. Peter Pan was always my favorite fairy," he laughed. "Believe in fairies. Believe in magic. Be open to help and open to love and kindness. And to love itself. Get outside of yourself and do something for others. Believe in the possibilities. Believe in yourself. Love yourself, be loving toward yourself, whatever that means for you."

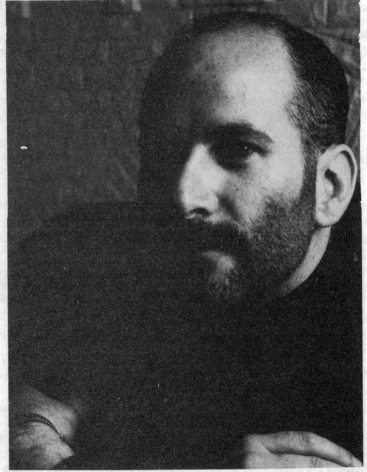

Cristofer Shihar.

Photo © 1988 by Daniel Adams.

CRISTOFER SHIHAR

"I'm proof that there's no right way or wrong way."

▨▨▨ I did something apparently quite rare in Los Angeles—I walked. Cristofer lived not far from where I was staying and, silly me, I decided not to bother with my rental car, since parking in West Hollywood is becoming as difficult as parking in the West Village.

When Cristofer opened the door he could see I was disoriented. "What's wrong?" he asked. I explained that everyone had stared at me. Cars had slowed to a crawl, pointing as I walked. Was I unzipped?

He laughed, for the first of many times, and patiently explained that the only people out on Santa Monica at this time of night are young hustlers. In fact, he explained, so unthinkable is it for a Los Angelean to be walking that police have taken to *arresting* the barely postpubescent boys they find walking Santa Monica Boulevard.

"You should be flattered," he said.

"What? That people thought I was hustling?"

"No," he smiled. "That people thought you were young."

Thus did we establish that we were both of the same seventies generation of gay men. When I interviewed Cristofer in September 1987, he was thirty-seven and I was thirty-two.

"You look vaguely familiar," I said. For those of us who've had thousands of sex partners, saying that someone looks familiar often carries with it the uncomfortable possibility that one might have had sex with the person and not quite remember having done so. I didn't think we'd had sex, but . . .

"You probably recognize me from the AIDS documentary which recently aired on national TV," he said.

Suddenly, it clicked. "Did you ride a motorcycle?"

"Yep. That was me. I weigh a lot more than I did in the documentary, though. Actually, I've been in two documentaries. It's weird. I did one four years ago and they updated it. They edited it in such a way that they faded out from my initial interview right into me today. And I saw that I went from this little thin person to a big blown-up person." He laughed. "But what felt awful was that everybody who'd been in the original documentary had died, except for me."

On that sad note, we began the interview in earnest. I asked him to tell me his story.

"I was diagnosed with Kaposi's sarcoma in November 1982. I had a swollen lymph node in my groin the size of an egg, which they removed and biopsied. I had KS in my stomach and lymph system. I started on alpha interferon as part of the first study program at UCLA during Christmas week of '82. First I started on low-dose intravenous interferon, with Sub Q, and two months later, I got high-dose, which was 92 million units a day every other week. That meant I was in the hospital for all of '83 and through March of '84. Then I decided I just couldn't take it anymore."

He lit up a cigarette. Seeing my startled expression, he said, "Yes, I've started smoking again. I quit smoking five years ago, and a couple of weeks ago I said, 'Oh, I can have just one cigarette. . . .'" He snorted: "What an asshole!"

I decided to ask him right off why he thought he had outlived so many others.

"Miracles happen. I'll leave it at that."

"No pattern, just a miracle?" I asked, trying to conceal my disappointment at finding yet another religious explanation for what I considered very hard work.

"No, no patterns. Basically, during the first couple of years and during the whole time I was getting treatments, everything I did was probably the exact *opposite* of what I should have done. I stayed high on cocaine the whole time I was getting interferon and I really didn't stop until a couple of years ago, when I was already in complete remission."

I was stunned, but secretly delighted, that someone who had broken all the New Age rules had managed to survive and thrive. In fact, I learned that Cristofer's spiritual rebirth had come *after* remission.

"Spiritually, I changed a lot. My life-style has changed drastically, but only after I was in remission. I didn't do any drastic changes in diet; I ate healthy food, but I didn't eat health food, if you know what I mean. I'm proof that there's no right way or wrong way.

"Surviving certainly wasn't my stated goal. It just happened. I mean, I never looked at the big picture and said, 'I'm going to survive' or 'I love myself the way I am.' I worked at it, but I didn't work at it. I did what I had to do to survive the day without looking at the long-range picture. I don't think you can focus on the long-range and survive."

I asked him what he meant by "drastically changed life-style."

"Before my diagnosis, I was into lots of partying. Lots of sex and lots of drugs—MDA, Quaaludes, cocaine—and alcohol, of course. Now all that's changed."

"Didn't anybody lecture you about doing drugs while you were getting interferon?" I asked.

"Yes and no. I mean, people *always* lecture. And I probably beat myself up more than anybody beat me up. The doctors, of course, didn't say 'Do coke,' but then again, they didn't say 'Don't do coke,' even though they had to know. They kind of said, 'Well, we don't know what's going on; you're doing fine, but cocaine's not good for you; but in good conscience, we can't tell you to stop.' Who knows? The cure might be some combination of interferon and cocaine," he joked, half-seriously. "I'm in remission. I guess I give interferon some credit.

"I believe in Western medicine," he said, but like other survivors, he went on to express a paradoxical disdain for Western drugs. "The only reason I took interferon was because at the time, it was a choice between that or chemotherapy. My best friend had died ten years ago from cancer and I watched chemotherapy destroy him worse than cancer. I had decided I would never do chemotherapy. After a while, I realized that what I was feeling so shitty from was the *interferon*, not AIDS. And when I finally stopped the treatments, I started feeling 100 percent better.

After interferon, I have never considered experimental drugs. Of course, it's very easy for me to say I wouldn't because I'm feeling so well. If I were sick, I might grasp for anything. I don't believe I would do any other drugs, though. I was offered AZT when they first started the trials, but I decided not to do it. I was doing well and saw no reason to take it."

He also has chosen not to take Bactrim or any other form of PCP protection. I gently tried to urge him to reconsider the need for prophylaxis. He listened politely but was noncommittal.

"As far as holistics go, I meditate and I'm very involved with Sally Fisher and the AIDS Mastery. Actually, my first contact with anything spiritual was a Steve Levine workshop I did in early '84, while I was still getting interferon. After coming back from that retreat, I did an overdose of Seconal. I think it was a little too heavy for a first encounter. It was five days in a *nunnery*. Then I discovered Louise Hay, and through her, I found the Mastery. That just brought everything together—all the reading I'd been doing and all the spiritual work."

He went to his bookshelf and pulled out a classic holistic guide to healing. "It essentially says, 'Don't eat meat and you'll be healthy and cure yourself of AIDS.' " He harrumphed. "I say that's bullshit! But that's only my opinion. I see so many people living in fear, trying to do the 'right' thing; and it's killing them because they're not doing what they feel is right. All they see is that they're doing something wrong and that's why they're sick.

"People are looking for somebody else to give them an answer to questions there aren't answers to. I believe there're some valid things in everything. The question is, What is AIDS here to teach us? Or maybe there is *no* spiritual reason for this; maybe it's just a virus."

He paused to sip his drink. "I feel that Louise Hay has changed her outlook drastically in the last year or so. Before, when people would start getting sick, they'd stop going, because when they'd go, it was like, 'Well, you're dying, so you obviously don't love yourself.' To me, that was the most absurd thing in the world. I mean, we're all going to die. That's part of the life cycle!"

Cristofer spoke about how different he was now. "I'd never done political work before, but AIDS politicized me. I was on the board of AIDS Project Los Angeles for two years, and I started a support group for people with AIDS."

I wondered if, with such a busy life, he had a lover. "I don't have one now, but I'm *always looking!*" he said, smiling.

"What about family?" I asked.

"I have a very small family. A couple of cousins have been supportive. My mom died two years ago and my dad has been dead for ten years. My brother, who I was fairly close with, was semisupportive. But when I went back East to visit, I wasn't allowed to see his kids because I might 'infect them.' This was in '83. That pretty much ended my relationship with my brother. For a long time, I had nothing to say to him."

Because of the terrible side effects from interferon, Cristofer had been forced to quit his job as a hairdresser. Fortunately, between disability and proceeds from a disability insurance policy that his aunt had taken out when he was a kid, he manages to get by.

"By and large, my friends have been supportive," he said. "And AIDS Project Los Angeles was *very* good to me. Actually, it gave me my whole support system at the time. Unfortunately, all the people that I got support from have all died since then.

"Actually, I was in the first support group they had for people with AIDS. It was interesting, but I hated it. I absolutely *hated* it. I didn't like sitting in a group talking about everything that was happening that was awful. It wasn't a *support* group; it was a bunch of scared people not knowing what to do. It eventually just disbanded."

Knowing or knowing of other long-term survivors also helped him get by. It made it possible for him to ignore the media campaign that promoted AIDS as 100 percent fatal. "Fatalistic reporting always affects me, but I realized, hey, they just don't know. AIDS hadn't been around long enough to say it would have a 100 percent mortality. I knew I wasn't dead, and I figured they were just exaggerating. Negative coverage affected me more then than it does now."

Because knowing other survivors helped him, Cristofer now feels a responsibility to be public as a long-term survivor. "I definitely feel the pressure to be public. I have that responsibility to myself and to others. But I've definitely experienced some jealously as a long-term survivor. I've been asked, 'Why are you alive and they're dead?' And you feel awful. I have no answer."

I asked him if he'd thought a lot about dying. One advantage of cocaine, he explained, was that it kept him from thinking about death. "I was too high; I wasn't realistic. I guess I thought I was going to die from AIDS, but with cocaine, I didn't really think about it. At this point, I'm still not sure I'm not going to die; it's just no longer important."

What advice would he give to someone newly diagnosed?

"Do whatever you feel like doing. There's no right way and no wrong way. If you feel something is going to work, it probably will. I don't think diet makes much difference, but that's only what *I* believe. Each person has to do what he believes in. I have people come up to me and say 'I wanna get high.' They know I got high and they're looking for approval. But I don't recommend it. On the other hand, I don't *not* recommend it. You've got to do things for yourself, not because somebody says if you don't do this, you're wrong—if you don't do this, you'll die. If they knew what to do, there'd be a lot more people alive, right? I say, live your life, don't live your death."

Even though we had just met, Cristofer shared his deeply personal vision of AIDS: "I believe that AIDS is here to awaken the world—to heal the planet. I look at AIDS as a second coming of the Christ spirit."

But after this bit of cosmic seriousness, he couldn't resist returning to a humorous analogy: "There's an old Jewish story that applies to AIDS. Right now, most United States citizens are saying, 'Oh, don't worry; the leak is in the *back* of the boat, and I'm in the front.' The message of AIDS is that the world had better come together to deal with this; only then will it be gone."

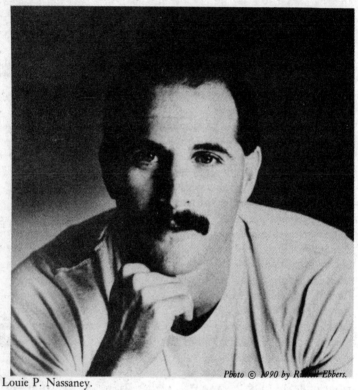

Louie P. Nassaney.

LOUIS NASSANEY

"Do what you want without guilt!"

▨▨▨ A Speedo-clad hunk sauntered by.

"There's one for you. Mmmm, *he's* cute," began Louie Nassaney as we spread out towels out on the sand of Venice Beach. "Of course, we PWAs don't *have* preferences anymore. We just take what's available," he joked.

"Any port in a storm," I opined. We had already fallen into the kind of instant intimacy that is so common among the soldiers in the trenches of this AIDS war. Peeling off his tank top and oiling his classically chiseled pecs, Louis pointed out that the view from this particular foxhole wasn't so bad.

Los Angeleno Louis Nassaney is one of the most famous long-term survivors. He has done many media appearances, culminating in a spread in the November 1985 issue of *People* magazine. He's also the star disciple of Louise Hay, New Age guru, whose merits and demerits are often hotly debated among PWAs.

"Let's see," he began with a tone that suggested he had told this story more than once. "Back in May of 1983 I was diagnosed with KS at UCLA. I haven't had anything else. The lesions seem to pop up when high stress comes into my life. I've been able to stay stable and my energy level is pretty good.

"My energy level basically corresponds to my diet. I dread Christmas and Thanksgiving: All that sugar just seems to throw me off. But," he quickly clarified, "if you're going to eat sugar, just don't have guilt! Have it and enjoy it. *Do what you do without guilt!* For instance, last night, I had french fries at the French Market. Have you ever had french fries there? They're these wonderful steak fries. And I put some salt on them and I just said, 'This is great! I have no guilt about these french fries. They taste great!' And it was absolutely wonderful. That's the key. If you choose to do other things, *just don't have guilt!*"

Speaking of food reminded Louie of the side effects he'd had while on interferon. "I had fifty percent loss of all my senses—my sight, my hearing, my touch, taste, and smell. Food tasted *terrible*. And I lost all my hair."

Although at the time he only had one KS lesion, Louie had entered an experimental interferon protocol at UCLA which he endured for seven months. "My KS lesion didn't disappear on interferon, but I didn't get any more. The doctors took me off the interferon because the lesion wasn't disappearing. I was willing to go through all the side effects, even though they were terrible: I was sleeping fifteen to twenty hours a day, and I was taking sixteen Tylenol a day to deal with my one-hundred-degree fevers.

"I was angry when they took me off interferon. They were going to put me on chemotherapy and radiation. It was at this point that I discovered my spiritual base."

I tend to curl my lip uncontrollably in the presence of New Age-y talk of spirituality; but something about Louie was simple, genuine, and direct.

"I had started going back to church and praying. I asked, 'What can I do to help myself?' And the message I felt from God was, 'Don't do anything more. You've already done your experiment.' And so I chose not to do anything else. And that's when I got connected with you-know-who: Louise Hay! In March 1984 I started listening to her tape "AIDS: A Positive Approach," and she relaxed me. Three months later, I met Louise.

"I had been reading about PWA Bobbi Campbell in San Francisco and was impressed because he was living with AIDS. I enjoyed those positive stories. Because I think that's what a person with AIDS needs: to see other examples. But Louise was the first person to tell me that I could live with AIDS."

Like other survivors, Louie's diagnosis motivated him to take an emotional inventory. His first decision was to end the relationship he was in.

"I had had a boyfriend for about three months when I was diagnosed. I decided that if I was going to do well with AIDS, I couldn't be in a relationship. I just needed to be by myself, to be alone. We talked, and I said, 'Listen, Billy, I have to go. I just have to go my way. I'm going to do well with this.' And he said 'Fine,' and that he would do everything in his power to support me. And we're still friends.

"Next, I dumped about 95 percent of my friends when I got diagnosed, because they were mostly party friends. When I got AIDS, I knew there was just no way that I could be around cocaine and Quaaludes and alcohol and the bar scene if I was going to get well. So I dumped them."

His diagnosis also drew him closer to his family. "We had a big family powwow. Everybody came. I told my parents and family that I was gay and that I also had AIDS, all on the same day. They responded with love and compassion, with tears and prayer and hope and more crying and more hugs."

He decided to quit his job managing his father's restaurant. Like many other survivors, he went on disability and pursued the new career of AIDS activist. "Now, I counsel people with AIDS all over the country. You should see my phone bill! I talk to people. And I'm involved in writing a book which Louise's publishing company, Hay House, will publish. I think it will be called *Life Is Worth Living, Even If You Have AIDS*. I want to dwell on the positives."

I asked Louie if he had any idea why he had survived so long after his diagnosis. He repeated a theme I had heard from other survivors: "Each one of us has his own recipe for living. All I can talk about is me. I try to eat well; I try to believe that I'm very strong. I do imagery and meditation and relaxation. I follow my own belief system. For example, I don't smoke cigarettes. But there are probably people with AIDS who are surviving while smoking cigarettes, and if they're happy doing it, fine."

Louie proceeded to express a contradiction I was to hear from several other survivors. Having tried experimental medications, he generally discouraged others from doing so. "I really think that the people who are living the longest are the people who are not going the so-called 'medical route.' It's the people who are willing to dive into life and do what they feel is right for them who are surviving."

Like other survivors, Louie spoke harshly about AZT. "I hear that if a healthy person takes AZT for five years, he will be dead. But," he continued, "if you're choosing AZT, see something positive in it. See some white light going through your body as you swallow it. Don't take the pill if you don't have the right attitude. If you take the pill and you're saying, 'This goddamned pill—I think it's no good,' then it won't work."

Louie much preferred to pursue anticancer therapies, such as carrot juice, suggested by holistic practitioners. I probed to see if he had completely abandoned Western medicine for New Age approaches to healing and discovered that, like many others, he'd struck a balance. "I get my blood work done every three months. I hope to God I never have to go back and even look at chemotherapy or radiation or interferon again. I believe in combining approaches. Western medicine should study people who are living with AIDS, especially us long-term survivors—people who've decided to live their lives, who have this incredible will to live, basically without medication. The long-term survivors are those who find a great *quality* of life, like yourself, myself, Cristofer, the Rev. Pieters. Look at the quality of the lives we lead!"

Louie reiterated his belief that it was important to spread the good news about AIDS. Because Louie has drawn strength from the example of others, he feels an obligation to stand up and be counted himself. "It comes with the territory. People who are living with AIDS have to speak up. It's our responsibility. I am healthy enough to help other people. God has given me this gift, so why not help other people? And when I help other people, they help me. I get a healing and they get a healing."

But Louie learned the hard way that one can overdo altruism. Louie learned to say no. "There's always my answering machine to screen calls, and there's always the word 'no.' I have no problem telling people that I can't help right now. Sometimes I just send them some of the stuff that's been written on me."

Saying no reminded Louie of the hard time he went through during the 1986 holiday season. "Have you noticed that lots of friends die around Christmastime? I was really depressed because lots of friends were really sick and dying. I wasn't working out. I started eating sugar and what I consider bad food and got *more* depressed. I was angry at the world and God, and boom, two lesions popped up. And then another week later, another lesion popped up.

"And I just said, 'Fuck it. Quit. Stop talking to them. You're depressed. You're angry. You need to be with yourself right now. You need time.' So I spent about two months with myself and had very quiet times. I remember running to Louise Hay. We both cried together for about a half an hour. A lot of her close friends had died too and she hurts a great deal, like we all do. And we both had an incredible release with crying."

After emerging from this depression, Louie decided to start what he called the "Healing Feeling" group for PWA followers of Louise Hay. "When I leave Louise's group, whether it's six people or six hundred, I always feel good, no matter what was talked about." Echoing the alcoholics Anonymous one-day-at-a-time sentiment, which runs deep throughout the PWA self-empowerment and New Age movements, Louie concluded: "If you take the healing feeling home and live it the next day, great."

Louie gave me an example of how diving into life can result in unexpected good luck. "I've been with my current lover for a year and a half. We actually met as a result of my *People* magazine profile. He was one of seventy people who wrote me. He was a very hurting young man. He's twenty-three. He said he hated himself for being gay, but he knew that he could help himself if he could talk to me. So we met, and here was this Italian super jock, with a deep voice, who was good-looking and had a body, and we went out to dinner and we just hit it off. I gave him Louise's book and taught him how to do mirror work. A week later, we met again and we made love—safe sex, of course. I never knew there was so much love. This is the first time I had had something from the heart."

He shook his head remembering how panicked he'd been the day he was diagnosed. "My doctor told me I'd be dead within three to six months. But in the back of my mind, I remember thinking '*Nothing* is 100 percent!' And I also thought, 'Well, if anybody can beat this, I can.' But to be honest, my own self-confidence was very low at the time."

Louie said he dealt with the media's campaign of gloom by simply not reading anything, or turning off the TV when an AIDS story came on. And he takes an aggressive stand against the fatalism whenever he speaks publicly. "I've been on several panels with a person from the AIDS Project Los Angeles. And when he speaks, it's all death and doom! He says AIDS is 100 percent fatal and everybody dies very fast. It's terrible.

"Then I follow him like some fairy godmother, or as I've been called before, the Mother Teresa of the West Coast. I talk about *wellness.* I mean, yes, people do die of AIDS; but there *are* people living with AIDS.

Louie and I were now preaching to each other, revving ourselves up to do battle against the doomsday attitudes we regularly encounter. "Living one day with AIDS is a survival. That's a miracle. That's what I tell people. If you feel good today, do something. Don't sit around and wait to feel better. Take advantage of feeling good."

Louie has avoided the hospice movement like . . . the plague. "I've stayed away from Shanti [an AIDS hospice group providing care to PWAs in the terminal stage of AIDS]. They're a death-and-doom/gloom group. They're changing, though. They've even begun to sponsor Louise, and they know she's gonna talk about living with AIDS."

Sometimes I worry that the huffing and puffing we survivors do about living with AIDS can contribute to denial about the seriousness of AIDS. Obviously, most people with AIDS do die of it. I asked Louie if he had thought about death. "Honey, like you, I've already *lived* my death. I've already had my death."

He got quiet for a moment and then said, "You know, everybody dies! So why think about it? Just go on living. If I get sick tomorrow and die from pneumocystis, I'll deal with it then."

Louie has also avoided the many PWA support groups that had sprung up around Los Angeles. "I don't go to the support group at APLA or Shanti, because they are *death* groups," he shuddered. "I didn't need to go to a group and cry my head off. I didn't need self-pity or sympathy at all. I need to be around people who share my belief that you can live with AIDS."

I asked Louie how he responded to the criticism I had encountered from many PWAs who said that Louise Hay's teachings imply that people who die from AIDS must not have loved themselves enough. He didn't bristle; he calmly explained, "Louise teaches people how to love themselves, and I think that's a gift. People try to turn that into some guilt factor. The New Age movement does teach that we are 100 percent responsible for our lives. But most people are only willing to accept responsibility for the good—if they win a car or get a wonderful boyfriend. But we are responsible for the bad that happens because of choices that we've made.

"Now I am not saying that people are *choosing* to get AIDS. I certainly did not choose to get AIDS. But I know that I created the circumstances which allowed this monster into my body. If I hadn't been doing drugs, cocaine and Quaaludes, and if I wasn't having all that rampant, wild sex, I would still have an immune system to take care of whatever would have invaded my body. Instead, I really ruined my immune system."

We talked about the thin line between blaming the victim and taking responsibility for one's healing. "I have seen people who have done Louise's method leave the planet," he said. "And it hurts. I'd like to say that Louise's method is the answer, but I can't. What I want to tell people who aren't doing well is that even if you're not doing well, you can always learn to feel good about yourself until that time for transformation comes.

"I have been with people who loved themselves right up until the moment of transformation. And I have been with people who have died blaming other people. I've been with people who have blamed the doctors, and blamed their chemotherapy and the goddamned doctors. But they *chose* chemotherapy. Nobody forced them. We've got to take responsibility. We can't start blaming other people for the decisions we've made. Take responsibility for your life, whatever happens, good or bad, and then move on."

This brought him back to his belief in the importance of having the right attitude. "Attitude is number one. I think that is the reason why the people I know are living with AIDS and doing well. I also recommend meditation, diet, nutrition, aerobics, working out. Sure, there are times when life creeps up behind you, and I hear my little ego say 'Unh-uh. You're gonna *die* from AIDS.' All I can say is you've got to start learning to live in the moment. Maybe everybody ought to get diagnosed with AIDS, if that's what it takes to realize what life is about. Live for the day and live for the moment. If you worry about the past and the future, you have no time left to live and enjoy life."

As we packed up our beach towels, he admired his tan and I complained about being sunburned. "It's immunosuppressive, you know," he joked.

"What isn't these days?" I asked.

Louie waxed philosophical. "I feel great. I'm happy. I'm wonderful. I have fun. And I enjoy life. If I get sick tomorrow, I'll deal with it. But today, I'm not sick. I am well and I feel great and I'm going to act like it."

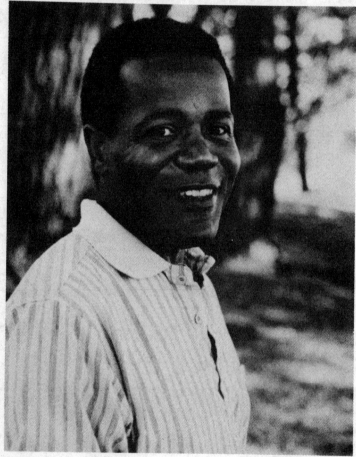

"A. J." Roosevelt Williams.

Photo © 1990 by Lanz Lowen.

"A. J." ROOSEVELT WILLIAMS

"It's about feeling like your life matters!"

▨▨▨ I met "A. J.," as he prefers to be called, thanks to the modern marvel of videotape. I had almost forgotten doing a documentary interview when a videotape of the final edit arrived in the mail. Absently, I put the tape on while ironing shirts. The segment following mine featured "A. J." Roosevelt Williams, an articulate forty-three-year-old black gay man who is a long-term survivor from Oakland, California.

I tracked him down and, after playing telephone tag, interviewed him by phone. We hit it off right away and, within minutes, he was thoughtfully answering the most shamelessly intimate questions.

Like so many of us, A. J. says it is difficult to pinpoint precisely when his AIDS saga began.

"As early as 1979," he recalled, "something was wrong with my immune system. I was coming down with bacterial pneumonias at least once a year, and sometimes twice. I had a low white count, swollen lymph glands, and unexplained bouts of itching."

Finally, in March 1982, A. J. (then thirty-five years old) checked into the New York Hospital for Joint Diseases and had a grueling battery of tests performed. He wasn't aware that the doctors were looking for AIDS. Instead, A. J. suspected that his health problems were related to the chronic hepatitis he'd had since 1975.

"AIDS just didn't register in my mind as anything I needed to be concerned about. But as a result of all the tests, they told me I had AIDS. I'd had what they told me were KS lesions for at least a year, maybe two, prior to that hospitalization, so technically, I may have had AIDS at least since 1981," he explained.

In June of 1982, A. J. moved back to the Bay Area. "Because I seemed to be so healthy otherwise, for a number of years, I preferred to think I only had ARC. But during that time, I continued to get bouts of bacterial pneumonia. And I began to have yeast problems—first on my fingernails and eventually in my esophagus. My T-cell count was steadily getting lower.

"At some point, though," he recalled, "it was obviously AIDS, not ARC. Recently, I developed MAI, an awful kind of tuberculosis for which I have to take five powerful antibiotics. Also, I have this gland in my groin which is swollen the size of a hard-boiled egg. They don't have a clue as to what it is.

"Besides AIDS, lots of things were happening all at once in my life," he said with wry understatement. "I lost my insurance in 1985 because TWA fired me. Once that happened, I was forced onto Medicare/Medi-Cal and Social Security. None of the doctors I was seeing would see me without cash payment or insurance, and none of them would take Medi-Cal. Fortunately, I had enrolled as a student at U.C. Berkeley so I now get medical care though the university," he said.

"I also had problems with Social Security. They arbitrarily cut off my payments. For three months I had no income. And that meant that I lost my home. Prior to this, a black AIDS agency in Oakland had made a commitment to my landlady to help pay my rent. But when the rent came due, they didn't pay it, and I was evicted. So for the last year and a half, I've kind of been wandering around, staying with my brother for a while, or with a friend in the city, and feeling rather homeless."

A. J. is amazingly resilient, even cheerful. I asked him how he has managed to be so optimistic through so much trauma.

"When they told me I had AIDS, I did not accept that it was the death sentence they were all telling me in so many words that it was. I just automatically felt that I might survive it. I wasn't naive enough about AIDS to say, 'No, I know *absolutely* I'm going to beat this.' But I just had this feeling inside that it didn't have to be fatal. I couldn't help feeling that some part of it was up to me, and if so, I was going to give it 100 percent of my efforts."

I asked him why he seemed to take his diagnosis so easily in stride. He paused to consider the question.

"I didn't immediately think that I had to accept AIDS as a death sentence because I'd already had horrible things happen and I'd somehow managed to fend *them* off.

"I'm the oldest of six illegitimate children brought up poor in the black ghetto in Oakland by a single parent living on welfare. I was pretty much brutalized as a child. I was molested by the husband of one of my mother's friends. And when I was twelve, I was molested by a Baptist preacher—

which was *truly* traumatic. The weird thing is, there was some part of me that wanted to be with a man. But I didn't know how to articulate that or even how to define it at twelve.

"I was getting all kinds of negativity about being a sissy. My mother beat me daily, and finally, when I was sixteen, she came after me with a butcher knife. I was taken from her and put in a foster home.

"It's strange," he recalled. "Even though I was beaten a lot and knocked around for being different, I grew up being everyone's sort of 'Black Hope.' I've always tried to survive in spite of my problems. Very early on I created an active public life as a way of making up for what went on at home. I was a Red Cross volunteer, Senior Class President, Student Body President, Alameda County Boy of the Year. You name it, I did it."

I asked A. J. why he had returned to the city where so many painful events had taken place. "I came back to California," he explained, "hoping I would find friends and family to connect with for support, but I didn't get much support for believing I could survive. My family essentially had nothing to do with me.

"I have a very strange family," he said, laughing good-naturedly. "We all live in the same town and yet nobody sees each other. One of my brothers lives right here in Oakland and I haven't seen him in eight years! I've been told that he has some issues around my being gay and around my having AIDS.

"But it's hard to say why we're all so distant. Maybe it's because my mother had told my brothers and sisters that I had left home because I was ashamed of the family. One of the things I'm hoping to resolve in my life is to talk with each one of my brothers and sisters to explain why I kept away. But it's hard because we've all kept away from each other.

"But my youngest brother, who is now a policeman, did make an effort," he said. "He would call once a month to see how I was. We were actually living together for a while after I came back to California. It's odd, after all these years of feeling like I had no family, to suddenly discover that I do indeed have a brother that really loves me.

"He has a daughter—*my niece,*" he said with obvious pride, "who is now four years old. My brother really makes an effort to make certain that I'm a part of her life. And I love him for that. And I think he genuinely loves me too."

I asked him if he had found knowing other people with AIDS to be helpful.

"I tried to connect with others in the beginning. I approached the Shanti Project twice when I came back to California, and twice they told me they weren't interested in helping me. My feeling is that it was because of racism, but it may just have been the particular individuals who happened to talk with me. Or maybe I was considered too healthy, 'cause at that time Shanti was mostly involved with helping people die. But if so, that wasn't made clear to me."

Eventually, A. J. did join a support group. "It was made up entirely of other men of color with AIDS and ARC. Everyone was either gay or bisexual. Unfortunately," he sighed, "I didn't find it very helpful. I was interested in living and doing all those things that would support living. Nearly everyone else in this group had accepted dying and did not see that there was anything for them to do to increase their chances. They admired me, and said so openly—that they really loved the fact that I was trying so hard. But they weren't willing to do it themselves.

A. J. has a theory about why the other men in his support group seemed to have given up.

"One of the issues I uncovered in myself was *internalized* racism. And I saw that as a problem for many gay black men, if not blacks in general. I wanted so much to find a place where I could talk that out and share with others and hear what it was for other people to have had that experience. But that was the real bugaboo. *Nobody* wanted to deal with that," he laughed.

"It had taken me a long time to understand that a lot of the loneliness that I had felt all my life was because I was a black man trying to fit into a white world where I wasn't really wanted. Only since getting AIDS have I realized how self-destructive some of the patterns I'd been involved in were. And as I looked at that more and more, I began to realize that it was probably true for many other people of color. I began to see how the drug problem in the ghetto has its roots in racism and in internalized racism.

"To give you an example of racism, when I came back to San Francisco with this AIDS diagnosis, San Francisco was paying more attention to AIDS than just about every other city. Every day on television there was something in the news. But I soon realized that whenever anything about AIDS was reported, it was always a gay white man. And even when they spoke of volunteers, it was always white people who were doing the volunteering.

"And to be honest with you, I started to feel jealous. I was watching these people become heroes and stars and I felt like I was being neglected. I realized that this must be true for other people too. Here we have black children in a ghetto who feel doubtful about a future to begin with. The world is saying to them, 'Just say no to drugs and make something of your life, but we're not going to show you any images of you as a hero.'

"And when I realized the hypocrisy in that, anger and resentment started to grow inside. Because I realized it's about feeling like your life matters! And if the world you live in continues to show you images which say that you don't matter—you don't count—that's going to influence how you feel about yourself and how you make choices in life."

A. J., ever the fighter, decided to act on his growing realization of the consequences of the myth that AIDS was only a white man's disease.

"I began to speak publicly as a black person with AIDS. And much of what I had to say addressed racism. I feel like AIDS is no accident. I can't help feeling that it is the result of how we've lived our lives as a people. AIDS to me is symptomatic of problems that have been there all along, even before AIDS came along. Mind you, I'm not saying that there's something wrong with being gay or wrong with being black that automatically makes you have AIDS. But I think any people who are oppressed—and I include in that group gay white men, Chicanos, and blacks—if you're oppressed long enough, you begin to internalize that oppression. You begin to act out your life in ways that are self-destructive, in ways that are now referred to as 'high risk behavior.' I felt that if we were ever going to deal realistically with AIDS, then we'd have to deal with the underlying problems that lead to having AIDS."

A. J. is particularly bitter about racism in the gay community. We both agreed that in a better world, white gay men who have themselves experienced the bitter sting of oppression for being gay would make an effort not to oppress others.

A. J.'s resilience in the face of overwhelming odds struck me as noble. As a gay man, I have felt that I've had to invent myself, with no role models to show me the way and in the face of powerful forces bent on convincing me that I am worthless because of how I love. I shuddered to think how much more difficult my own life would have been if the additional burden of racism had been added. A. J.'s willingness to confront problems head-on humbled me.

"It angers me that the gay community continues to be as racist as it is. Recently, I passed a very popular photo developing store in the Castro area. They had hundreds of pictures in the window from the Halloween festivities, and *not one photo was of a person of color!* That *scares* me!"

He got quiet for a moment, as if he was processing a painful memory. "I wasn't too aware of racism in the gay community before. All my life I've tended to be the only black person in most groups and it wasn't an issue for me. But at this point in my life, it is.

"This may seem strange to say, but I think a lot of the problems between me and other black men was a cultural thing. Despite the fact that I came from abject poverty, I've somehow managed to have enough cultural experiences to become very different from most other black men. I've lived around the world. I speak several languages. I played viola from the time I was a little child. That doesn't make me better than other black men, nor did I ever see it that way. But when it came to sharing interests and talking about things, I rarely found a black person who had had those kinds of experiences in common with me.

"All my life it's been easier for me to deal with white men. Not to mention that the society that I lived in kept telling me that white men are what are beautiful. Now, I think white boys are cute! I *love* 'em," he giggled. "But I was having this experience of not liking myself very much.

"I don't want to be where I'm not wanted, and I don't want to want people who don't want me. I think I'm a loveable person and I think I deserve a chance too, and I want to go to those places where there is a chance.

"I live with a certain amount of anger," he said. "The challenge for me is learning how to use that anger constructively. There's lots to be angry about."

I asked him what his approach to treatment had been and how he felt about alternative approaches to healing. I was delighted to discover another AZT heretic.

"I've tried to arm myself by learning as much as I could about AIDS and my treatment options," he said. "My attitude is one of being very suspicious of Western medicine. I have a reputation among my doctors for being . . ." He paused to choose his word carefully. "I'm pretty . . . self-willed," he said, laughing.

"I cannot be made to do things I don't want to do. And I did not want to do AZT. I finally gave in in November 1989, but I couldn't tolerate it at all and stopped after two weeks. You can't cure anyone with a poison, and AZT is obviously a poison on some level because of the toxic things it does. And with my history of liver disease, I have to be very careful about drugs.

"Actually, I've been *gaining* weight over the whole eight year period," he complained, "while everyone else I know with AIDS is losing weight. So I've felt that maybe what I'm doing is working; maybe I should just trust my instincts."

I asked him if he had taken any drugs besides AZT.

"I've been doing aerosolized pentamidine for about a year and a half," he said. "I've taken Bactrim on and off for the various bacterial pneumonias I had. But through most of this the only real medicine I took was ketaconazole for thrush. Everything else was nutritional: garlic pills, vitamin C, germanium. There was a while there when I was actually drinking food grade hydrogen peroxide. I did egg lipids for a long time and couldn't tell if it helped or hurt, so I let it go. I try things and if they work, I stick with them; if not, I move on."

"What about holistics?" I asked.

"I think Western medicine is really good at certain kinds of things, mainly diagnosis. But there are lots of things that affect health that Western medicine doesn't take into consideration. My rule has been, 'Beyond a wholesome discipline, be gentle with thyself.' I don't want to stick to anything so rigidly that the very act of sticking to it makes you a miserable person. Most of my adult life, I've supplemented my diet with vitamins and herbs. I try to eat a balanced diet that does not include dairy products, sugar, or highly refined or processed foods. And I avoid red meat. But occasionally, I break all my own rules, like I did at Christmastime when I let myself have some wine. That was the first time in two years that I'd had any alcohol and it was *wonderful.*"

"Aside from diet," I asked, "have you tried any of the other alternative approaches popular among PWAs?"

"I think there's a lot that's true in alternative systems: visualization, body work, vitamins, nutrition, and diet. I find meditation very helpful. But I don't agree with Louise Hay; I don't think that self-love comes from repeating affirmations. I think you have to really dig deep and look inside and work on those places that contribute to why you don't love yourself."

I asked him whether he had found comfort in religion or spirituality.

"All my life I've told people that I'm an *extremely* religious person . . ." he paused for dramatic effect, "but one who doesn't believe in the *church.* I can't help feeling that much about the church has contributed to the problems that we face with AIDS—especially black churches. But I think Christ had incredible lessons to teach us about what's important: loving each other, loving ourselves, and being active about that.

"I made a very conscious decision at seventeen to leave the Baptist church because of its stand on homosexuality. Over the years, I've explored other possibilities. I've spent some time studying Vedanta and yoga and Zen Buddhism and Tibetan Buddhism; but I never felt like I could commit to any of them either."

I asked A. J. whether he had any goals for the future. His answer was quick: finding a lover and getting his degree in mathematics.

"I still desire intimacy and closeness. Since being diagnosed, I've had two disastrous affairs. I'm still very much open to having a lover relationship, but I'm doing nothing to bring it about. Lots of things that I want to have happen for me I don't feel will happen until I have a home. But

I'm realistic; I think my chances of getting a lover are pretty reduced. We live in a youth culture and I'm in my mid-forties. I have AIDS, and I think most people, including gay men, are at some level AIDS-phobic. So I think it's going to be difficult. But I don't think it's impossible."

I told him that he was one of the most elligible PWA bachelorettes that *I* knew. He laughed.

"I've got a year to go to complete my degree in mathematics," he said proudly. "To be honest with you, when I decided to go back to school, it was mainly about wanting to have a future. It's hard to explain. When someone would say to me, 'Oh, what are you doing next week? Or next month?' I truly drew a blank. That might have been part of being in a state of shock over the diagnosis. I don't know. But I just knew in a very conscious way that I didn't know how to think about the future. Once I enrolled in school, the very act of enrolling was an act of faith that I *had* a future.

"I realize that in a sense, going back to school was naive. I mean, what will be my chances of getting a teaching job. I'm a black, openly gay man with AIDS in his middle forties! What are the chances anyone is going to give me a job teaching mathematics in white America?" he asked rhetorically.

I asked A. J. to describe how AIDS has changed him.

"Shortly after being diagnosed, I examined what my life had been—the kind of choices I had made, how I'd lived my life. I did this out of the belief that some part of my having this disease was my responsibility. I don't mean that in the sense of feeling like I caused myself to have AIDS, but I feel like some part of how I am made it possible for this disease to come into my life. So I looked at that.

"And what I saw was the numbers of years I had hung out in gay bars desperate for affection. And I thought about the money I had spent on alcohol and cigarettes and marijuana. I was waiting for something to happen that never happened. It may be a peculiarity of mine that I can look at my life that way and not beat myself up for it—and I know people may think this sounds like I'm blaming myself—but I'm not. I just had this feeling that to a degree I could be responsible, then to that same degree I could have control and could influence my chances of living."

In all my interviews, I'd not heard a more succinct statement of the empowerment that can come from taking responsibility for one's choices.

A. J. continued: "I still see that I'm growing as a person and there are more changes for me to make. Death has not been a major preoccupation in my mind throughout this crisis, until last November when I became very ill. Even then I didn't think about dying, because when problems come up, my focus tends to be: What can I do to resolve this? How do I get over this problem? I never think of any problem as signaling the end. I'll probably go through a period where I may feel frightened about death. But right now I don't."

I ended our interview by asking A. J. the same question I'd asked every other survivor: What advice would he give to someone who had just been diagnosed?

"Oh, boy," he gasped. "I wish I had a *week* to think about it before I had to answer." After a long silence, he said "I have the feeling that the success of our lives is really dependent upon the degree to which we can accept the truth about our own lives. I mean being *painfully* honest with yourself about who you are, what you are. I really think that's the key. To the degree to which you're able to face yourself honestly and face life honestly, to that degree do you give yourself a chance to survive. And you can't give in to fear. I think part of the reason I've survived so long is that I didn't respond to AIDS with fear.

"In a strange way," he observed, "I am happier today than I ever was, in spite of having AIDS. Even though my circumstances are worse, I feel happier because of what I've learned and what I've seen. There's a kind of confidence that comes only with the truth; even when things are horrible all around you, you still feel empowered because you know your own truth. I'm talking about the truth that's inside of you. It's not some external vision with the clouds parting and messages written in the sky," he laughed.

"Diet, nutrition, mental attitude, and all that is also important, but if you tell yourself the truth, all those things will come automatically and you'll know where they fit and what to do about them. But it all begins with somehow first coming to terms with the truth of who you are. That would be my advice."

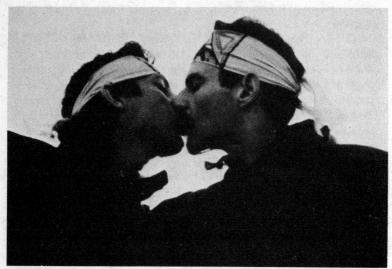

Michael Callen, left, and Dan Turner.

Photo © 1986, 1987 by Jane Rosett.

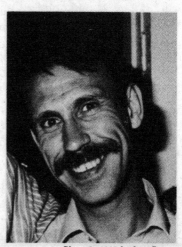

John Lorenzini.

Photo © 1987 by Jane Rosett.

DAN TURNER AND
JOHN LORENZINI

"See it as a challenge and an opportunity."

▨▨▨ It was like a veterans' convention: Dan Turner, John Lorenzini, and I together in Dan's sunny backyard perched high in the Castro hills drinking cranberry juice and club soda instead of the beer that is more traditional at such gatherings. Dan Turner is probably the most famous long-term survivor in San Francisco—maybe even in the world. John Lorenzini is not far behind him in fame and survival time. When we were reunited in October 1987, we joked that added together, Dan's five-year survival, my four and a half years, and John's four years totaled thirteen and a half AIDS years!

We had all been very active in AIDS politics, and specifically in the messy politics of the People with AIDS self-empowerment movement. I had met Dan at the historic 1983 AIDS conference in Denver, which is considered the founding moment of that movement. At the time of our interview, John Lorenzini was co-chair of the National Association of People with AIDS, an organization which grew out of the Denver conference.

Each rolled his eyes to heaven when asked to put his individual "AIDS 101" down on tape for posterity. We had each been asked to tell our sad tale so many times that, we joked, it would probably be more fun for each of us to tell the other persons' stories instead of our own.

"I noticed my first lesions in December 1981 and was officially diagnosed with Kaposi's sarcoma on February 12, 1982," Dan began. "I was the first case of KS and AIDS my doctor had seen. He was a holistic doctor and he recommended that I 'look into myself.' " Dan laughed, recalling how naive we had all been back then. "My holistic doctor was wondering whether gay men were getting this disease because of low self-esteem or something, and so he recommended that I 'look into my feelings.' He also urged me to go in the direction of alternative therapies. Although he was gay, he has since," Dan deadpanned, "given up medicine and gotten married to a woman."

Dan then started going to Dr. Marcus Conant, soon to be regarded as one of the foremost AIDS experts in San Francisco. "The University of California Medical Center put me through a battery of tests at Dr. Conant's urging: a lymph node biopsy, colonoscopy, endoscopy, and a CAT scan. Everything was negative. He sent me to the new AIDS clinic being run by Dr. Paul Volberding at San Francisco General. Ron Carey, who turned out to be another long-term survivor, and I were the first two patients to attend the clinic." Dr. Volberding advised Dan to avoid aggressive, immunosuppressive chemotherapy. Dan instead chose to do vinblastine, a popular chemotherapy considered less toxic, once a week for two months. To his immense joy, the lesions stopped progressing.

Like many PWAs, Dan has always tried to strike a balance between allopathic medicine and holistics. While on chemotherapy, he began acupuncture. "During treatments," he recalled, "I would meditate and concentrate on creating an energy flow to eradicate the cancer cells. I had the image that my cancer was due to a blocked immune system."

Dan got some important advice from another holistic practitioner. "He said I could cure myself through diet, acupuncture, and self-expression. He knew I was a writer, so he encouraged me to purge my blockages through writing. That's how I got into public speaking, appearing on panels and at forums as a publicly identified PWA. It was really therapeutic; by talking about AIDS, I felt in control of it."

Like me, Dan met an important role model who preached survival at a very crucial point in his diagnosis. "Bobbi Campbell was the first person to go public with AIDS. He actually had a regular column in the newspaper. The very first week of my diagnosis, he came over. We sat in my living room and talked. Bobbi was wearing his little yellow 'Survive' button and we showed each other our lesions and held hands on the sofa. He explained that the tests I was about to have were 'a breeze.' He made me feel comfortable. He was very positive about our chances for survival and gave me a lot of confidence."

Dan used a curious form of denial to ease himself into the full knowledge that he had AIDS. "My diagnosis was of cancer, not AIDS. That was an important distinction for me. Although I was still upset to be told I had cancer—it was like the death of little Nell," he joked, "I remember thinking in the back of my mind, 'Well, some people beat cancer. Maybe I will.' And I knew from a prior experience with hepatitis that if I fell into a negative attitude, I would die. So while the doctor was explaining KS to me, I was silently telling myself, 'Don't pretend to be more sick than you are.'

"But later that year, when the word 'AIDS' came out, I felt like I had gotten a second diagnosis. But at that point, my cancer had stabilized and the acronym 'AIDS' didn't come out until the fall of '82. Cancer was the worst thing anybody could say to you before AIDS. And I told myself that's what I had—cancer. And the stories of people getting over cancer were a little core of hope. Sometimes that's all you need."

The novelty of AIDS made Dan a guinea pig for doctors who were trying to understand the disease. He ended up quitting his word-processing job. "I was a star case in the beginning. Everybody wanted a biopsy or a blood donation. Everybody wanted their own pound of flesh. There was so much testing going on that I couldn't keep my job."

Dan began a new career as a PWA public speaker. In early May 1982, after nine treatments of chemotherapy, Dan ran in the grueling Bay-to-Breakers race. San Francisco gay activist Cleve Jones asked Dan to address a crowd that had assembled on Castro Street. In the two minutes allotted to him, he spoke simply and directly about his illness. He described KS and his treatments and announced that he'd just completed the race. "I remember that a cheer went up. I guess they liked the idea that I was fighting it. I didn't tell them," he confided, laughing, "that I had joined the race midway."

But his optimism was tempered by a realistic sense of how serious AIDS was. "I was thinking about the possibility of dying. I remember my first TV interview, the guy came over and stuck a microphone in my face and said, 'How does it feel to know you'll be dead in two months?' It hit me; I hadn't put a number on it before. There's a long gap in the interview where I said nothing. I assumed they'd cut out that gap. But that's exactly what they showed—they showed my stunned look and held it through the long gap."

Gradually, Dan began to experience the stigma of AIDS. "I had met someone in San Diego. The first time I visited him, right before leaving for the beach, I blurted out that I had KS. Although he let me visit again, he made me sleep on the couch."

After completing standard chemotherapy for his KS, Dan and his friend Ron Carey were offered the chance to enter one of the first interferon protocols. "I remember that Dr. Volberding walked into the room and pointed first at Ron and then at me and said, 'You get the high dose and you get the low dose.' Ron had terrible side effects: chills, fevers. He had to get in a tub of ice to cool down. Being on low dose, I had virtually no side effects, aside from flulike symptoms and generally lower energy."

Dan had entered the AIDS treatment treadmill. For five consecutive days a week, one week on and one week off, Dan got interferon injections. He remains on interferon to this day, although the schedule is now one week on, two weeks off. "On interferon, the lesions that I had became inactive and some faded away. My lesions became inactive and essentially went away by the end of '82. And it's remained the same. The only other problems I've had are shingles, some other annoying skin infections, and a bizarre cough that comes and goes."

I was startled to discover that Dan is not on pneumocystis prophylaxis. I launched into my standard sermon about the wisdom of PCP prophylaxis. I asked Dan whether or not he was taking AZT. He told me that despite pressure to take AZT, he had originally resisted. He has since given in to the pressure several times, although he never remains on AZT for long. "Aside from interferon, I haven't tried the other therapies. I haven't felt the need. Essentially, my system's been stable for more than five years. The cancer is in remission. But I do have to watch my stress levels. The shingles outbreak came during a period where I was really stressed out and not able to express my anger. But currently, I feel well."

As Dan paused in his tale, I tried to recall if this was the first time the three of us had ever been alone together. I'd been alone with Dan and I'd been alone with John, but we'd never all actually sat down to compare AIDS horror stories. The interview for this book had provided the excuse we needed to get together.

John Lorenzini, who was living in San Francisco when he was diagnosed with KS in 1983, had recently returned from Salt Lake City, where he had moved in 1986 to start an AIDS education organization.

Why Salt Lake City? "It's a long story. I was born in Denver and raised in a small town in western Nebraska. While in Vietnam, I converted to the Mormon faith. I came back from Vietnam and went to Brigham Young University. But I was excommunicated over the issue of my homosexuality. Then I found out that someone I knew had been excommunicated from the Mormon Church when he was diagnosed with AIDS. And he basically walled himself off and chose to die; he didn't last very long. That motivated me to move back to Salt Lake City to see if I couldn't change some attitudes."

"I think both John and I have felt a responsibility toward warning the community," said Dan. "Going public with our diagnosis was a way of confronting AIDS; we took control by talking about it.

"People come up to me and say, 'You're so public! What about your family and friends?' " he continued. "They give you the impression that you really should be embarrassed or ashamed. Well, if you start listening to everybody, you'd crawl back in the closet. And like John said, I know friends who did exactly that, and they died—like *that*," he said, snapping his fingers for emphasis.

"We have to reclaim our lives," John said. "I think that first of all, people have to accept AIDS into their lives. It's not a punishment; it's not a condemnation; it's not a judgment; it's simply a fact of life. You can't panic; you have to ride with it and be very careful. If you were to throw me in the water, I would drown if I panicked. But if I relax, I have a chance of floating and surviving."

John's careful, reasoned approach to AIDS extends to his approach to healing. For example, he has chosen not to take AZT, despite the enormous pressure to do so. He said he had seen too many people get sick from AZT and felt he was already stabilized. "The attitude I share with my doctor is, why fuck with success," he said. "I don't panic about treatment decisions. I thoroughly review the various treatment options, look them over, check out their side effects, watch what other people do and see what happens to them. I stand back. If there's ever a successful treatment for AIDS, I'm sure I'll find out about it.

"Both John and I respect traditional medicines," said Dan. "But we also both are open to alternative therapies. There's a certain amount of trust that goes into it."

Both count themselves lucky that Dr. Volberding has been their physician. "He's open to alternative therapies. He works *with* us instead of telling us what to do."

"With my doctor, decisions are *joint* decisions," John said. "My doctor exudes a sense of calmness and relaxation which you pick up; it makes you feel good, and that's where healing begins."

"In the twentieth century, we all want an instant cure. We've been trained to think that way. But patience is what's necessary for healing to take place. The body wants to live, wants to heal itself; but I have seen people rush into harsh treatment too soon and overwhelm their bodies," Dan warned.

"And even with experimental protocols," explained John, "the people who are still alive today are alive because they got off the protocol when they started to see serious side effects. They didn't wait for their doctor to say, 'Gee, you know, you're doing badly and it looks like you're going to die.'"

John had been using alternative chemotherapeutic drugs to treat his KS, but "when I started having the tingling sensations which precede peripheral neuropathy, I said, 'Stop. I don't want any more of this.' You're the one living inside your body; you're the one who should be calling the shots.

"Looking around, I see people who panicked and jumped into drug treatment protocols, or people who continued to use recreational drugs or abuse their bodies. They disappear fast. And the same thing happens if you don't take care of your mental and emotional health. You have to accept that you're in the water. You have to begin to tread water and to be very careful to take care of both your mental and physical health."

"When I feel myself beginning to panic," Dan said, "I visualize the idea of eradicating and replenishing my blood. I sometimes visualize my KS like shredded wheat, crumbling. I had seen a *National Geographic* photo of a dead cancer cell and thought it looked like shredded wheat. I feel that the virus and I can live together; we can coexist."

"I also exercise to reduce stress," Dan said. "It's also an important part of one's self-image to feel sexually attractive." His humpy, lumberjack physique confirmed his commitment to exercise.

"I know that both Dan and I have gone back to dating and doing everything that we did before," said John. "It's important to participate in life to its fullest. Of course, that means safe sex and taking care of our bodies. The key is to go on with your life, regardless of what AIDS is doing."

AIDS is only the latest crisis in John's life. His life story is filled with instances where he'd had to triumph over a difficult situation. He'd survived a life-threatening childhood illness, several close calls as a soldier in Vietnam, and a serious accident where he was pinned under a forklift that had fallen off a barge into an ice-cold river. But of all his struggles, the most difficult had been accepting his gayness.

"I'm from Nebraska. When I discovered my homosexuality back in '65, I quickly learned that they locked you up in a penitentiary as a felon, or locked you away in a mental hospital and subjected you to electroshock therapy. I really wrestled with my gayness. But I had a sort of daydream/ vision where I realized that I have this guardian angel that's been protecting me all my life. I've been through several very close, near-death situations. I've been through Vietnam, and many times when I should have died, I didn't. I survived! I believe that there's something very powerful, supernatural, protecting me. I got to meet this guardian angel after I was diagnosed with AIDS. Basically, what I understand from the vision is that this angel who is protecting me is somebody from a past life, from ancient Greek times, who was my lover. And regardless of what society thinks, love is something that endures and is respected by the Creator. I believe that my gayness is a gift. It's a gift that's difficult and brings responsibility, but I try to make the most of it.

"I believe that homosexuality and AIDS are some of life's toughest courses to take," John continued, "but if you really hang in there and sweat it out, you will be a phenomenally better person in the end. And I believe that when you leave this earth, you take not just the spirit of who you are, but you take your experiences with you too.

"AIDS is nothing to be ashamed of. If you can see it as a challenge and an opportunity, the question becomes, What do I want to do about it?"

"I've always prayed daily to keep up my spiritual life," Dan said. "And I've used some Christian imagery in my visualizations."

One consequence of being so involved in the PWA self-empowerment movement is that one has to endure the deaths of so many new friends. The emotional effects of all that death are profound. "The first death that really got to me was Bobbi Campbell's death in August of '84," Dan recalled. "I realized that I had never cried about my cancer, about AIDS, about any of it. But I cried for fifteen minutes solid when I heard Bobbi had died. I remembered him wearing his 'Survive' button.

"I feel peer pressure to be a survivor—to be a leader, and not let AIDS get me," Dan said. "When Bobbi died, I kept thinking to myself, where will we find another Bobbi? Bobbi was not only fighting for himself; he was fighting for all of us. And when he went into battle, he was carrying the standard for all of us. And then suddenly he was gone. And we realized that if we were going to go forward, we'd have to do it ourselves— hopefully with some others beside us too. When Bobbi died, I released all the tears inside me that had built up: being sorry for myself, being sorry for the fact that I had never cried. I just let myself go."

Both John and Dan suffered another devastating blow when *another* Bobby died: long-term survivor and PWA activist Bobby Reynolds. "A year after Bobby Reynolds's lover died," Dan said, "actually, on the *anniversary* of his lover's death, Bobby started to decline. He seemed to have lost his fighting spirit. Since he'd had minimal KS for over four years, it freaked me out that the death of his lover could have such an emotional impact on him. He had been so active: He'd been president of the San Francisco PWA group; he was active in the National Association of People with AIDS. But on the anniversary of his lover's death, he started to decline and eventually died. It struck me that he *decided* to die."

We wondered aloud whether Bobby's intense association with Shanti, an AIDS hospice group, had played a roll in his downturn. "I don't know whether it was the counseling of Shanti or just the fact that he'd been with Shanti for so long, but he did seem to make a decision to die," Dan mused.

Dan's talking about Bobby Reynolds's death reminded me about a postcard that I had gotten from Bobby. "I will be leaving you. . . ." it said. I remembered thinking he had given up.

"He even sent out a form letter announcing that he wanted to be remembered whenever we saw a rainbow," John reminded us.

"Now, Ron Carey couldn't have been more different," said Dan. "He was in the hospital twice a year for the last five years. He had KS and got PCP three times. He was in a coma last fall. Every time he was in the hospital, he pulled himself out. He rallied, because he had something to do: He had a Caribbean cruise planned, he had Mardi Gras to go to, or the Russian River, or the gay rodeo. He always had something he wanted to do and to live for. But he had the *worst* luck with treatments. Time and again he rallied. Even though he was thin and yellow, he rode in the gay pride parade in June. He loved life. Finally, this spring, he just dropped dead, essentially."

We were all momentarily silent, processing the enormity of our collective grief. "We've lost so many of the survivors. . . ." Dan muttered. "Paul Castro, with his wonderful sense of humor. I can still see him in the '83 gay pride parade, wearing a tutu and leaping the entire length carrying a sign that said 'A Leaper, not a Leper.' "

AIDS deaths seem to come in waves, and there had recently been a virtual tidal wave of AIDS deaths. "The accumulation of deaths, both of the long-term survivors and close personal friends, has been an emotional strain for me," moaned Dan. "I've just gotten numb. The entire board of the PWA Coalition died this year, except for two of us. And then David Summers died in New York, and Amy Sloan in Indiana. I mean, thanks to the fact that the PWA movement is now national, we're no longer just dealing with local deaths. If you sit and think about it, and begin counting the deaths, you go nuts. You have to go back to the one-day-at-a-time philosophy and think, well, what can I do about today?"

Wanting to cheer us up, I suggested that we talk about *l'amour*. But for Dan and John, this topic wasn't much happier than the one we'd just been discussing.

"My love life has been a series of disasters," John said. "I had a relationship in '81 that broke up in '83 when I was diagnosed with AIDS. I've dated many people since then, and many have been PWAs and PWARCs. But they push me away, partly because I'm doing well and they're often not. They get very angry. So relationships have been a problem."

"In October of '82 shortly after I was diagnosed," Dan recounted, "I met this guy from Oakland. Before we had sex, I literally proposed marriage to him in the car. And he said, 'Well, let me think about it.' I told him, 'Well, you'd like a relationship and I'd like one. I'd like to be your lover.' It was just very cut-and-dried, direct. And he came back to me a little later and said, 'Yeah, I'd like to have a relationship; let's do it.' "

In medieval heterosexual courtship, the next step would have been to seek the permission of Dan's parents. But in the gay world in the age of AIDS, the next step was to meet Dan's doctor. Dr. Volberding talked to the two of them together about what they could do sexually, and then he talked to Dan privately. Dan's new lover had had his T-cells tested. "His ratio was like a *straight* man's!" Dan exclaimed. "So he knew he was healthy. So after our little talk with the doctor, we started our relationship and started having sex.

"And it was really a big surge of positive energy for me. He was very supportive. I was overwhelmed—not just to find someone willing to have a relationship with someone with AIDS, but overwhelmed at finding somebody in San Francisco who wanted to have a *relationship.* Come to think of it, though, he did live in Oakland. . . ." Dan joked.

"We always used condoms. But as the years went by, when he would take me to the hospital, he would see people with AIDS getting worse. First, he told me, 'I can't take you to the hospital anymore.' And the media began making a big impression on him; he was getting nervous. He started taking more vitamins than me! He was reacting more and more to the sensationalism of the press. It began to impact on our relationship. It got to the point where he was afraid to jack off because he might have cuts on his hand. So, after two years of bliss, because of the reports about saliva and all the deaths, it became too much for him. After three years, he broke up with me.

"I was *devastated.* We're friends now, but it was painful. Since 1985, I've been dating again. But the world was a different place; we were several years into AIDS. Another guy I was dating eventually also freaked out about AIDS. Now, when I date, I'm never quite sure whether AIDS is an issue, so I usually ask. And usually they deny that it has anything to do with AIDS. But in the back of my mind, something says, 'AIDS *does* make a difference. . . .' "

John disagreed. "I don't think it's made any difference at all for me. Because I can look back, I've always worked around my options. I once had a boyfriend who was triplegic and we just worked around it. I've just worked around AIDS as well. Besides, there are more and more people with AIDS to choose from. I mean, we're not such an exclusive club anymore," he said, laughing.

On that cheerful note, we ended our interview and got down to the serious business of discussing the latest intrigue in the AIDS activist movement.

"LELA"

"Fuck you, fuck you! To spite you, I lived!"

⊠⊠⊠ I didn't want to publish a book about long-term survivors that didn't include a profile of a woman surviving with AIDS. Sadly, available data indicates that women with AIDS tend to die much more quickly than gay men, and in particular, women of color whose risk factor is IV drug use tend to die very quickly. The median survival time listed in the first CDC study on New York City survival trends was a mere six months. I decided to abandon my arbitrary three-years-or-more cutoff and include this profile of a feisty female survivor who shows every sign of eventually surpassing the three-year mark—and beyond.

I met "Lela" (not her real name) at a National Association of People with AIDS conference held in Dallas in the fall of '87. Lela describes herself as "a former IV drug user" and "a lesbian—even though I have slept with men." When I interviewed her in the fall of 1989, this feisty woman was planning what she dubbed a "Fuck you, I've survived" celebration. Though she continues to be plagued by serious health problems, she has every intention of surviving AIDS.

It's hard to pinpoint precisely when Lela earned a diagnosis of full-blown AIDS, since a suspected bout of PCP was treated presumptively and successfully in February 1987. Having survived full blown AIDS for at least two years at the time of our interview, she had already survived nearly four times longer than the six-month median survival probability for women with AIDS.

Lela is a role model for many women with AIDS. Although she is publicly identified as a woman with AIDS, and has been extremely politically active, she wants to retain some degree of privacy. In an attempt to conceal her identity, I have changed some of the details in the story that follows. However, the essence of Lela is conveyed in the following interview.

▣ The most frustrating aspect of being a woman who has AIDS, Lela explained, is that everyone expects you to have AIDS in the same way that men do. "Everyone's image of AIDS is the emaciated, Dachau concentration-camp-survivor look. In fact, most of the women with AIDS I know are very large, like me—*robust,* as I would say. And the infections we get aren't always the same ones men get, so doctors often don't look for AIDS in women. And the reality is, there are a lot of women out there who you'll be sitting next to thinking they're fine, but I know them to be sick.

"I started shooting heroin when I was fourteen and did a lot of drugs as a child, so I knew that I was in a high-risk category. From '76 to '83, I didn't shoot drugs anymore, but I still did a lot of other drugs. And my life was pretty normal. Then in '83, I started shooting drugs again and my life went up and down. My drug of choice was heroin. I did fix in shooting galleries, but a lot of times I was able to cop drugs and go home to fix," she explained.

Lela periodically went off drugs on her own, without entering treatment programs. "In early 1984, I got clean again, and I stayed clean for six months. And then, when I was visiting New York in 1985, I went back out and stayed out in the East Village shooting drugs for about two months."

"Of course I'd *heard* about AIDS, but it didn't connect. Even in New York in 1985 we knew people were dying, but that knowledge wasn't as pervasive as it is now. And I had also not started to lose friends like I have now. I mean, in 1985, you didn't have AIDS Incorporated like we do now, so in the back of my mind, I only vaguely thought about AIDS. At this time, I was shooting drugs with two men who I presumed to be gay, though we were also having sex. And AIDS didn't really matter."

Even though she's been completely off recreational drugs for years, Lela rails against the stereotypes that most people have of IV drug users. She explained that not all IV drug users are suicidal and indifferent about their lives and their health, and that many IV drug users lead more or less normal lives and don't fit the classic stereotype of the junkie nodding out on the street corner.

"I was living in a car outside a flophouse, and I was doing drugs, but my life wasn't miserable. I wasn't unhappy. I was just doing what I was doing, and it was important to me at the time. If I judge what I was doing then from where I am now after four and a half years of sobriety, then I just beat myself up. But then, it was just that I couldn't find a handle. I was just doing what I knew to cope. It's not always like what you see on TV: the black junkie with the runny nose who's stealing their old lady's pocketbook or out on the street robbing people. There's a lot of people who keep it together who still shoot drugs. They've generally got a place to stay, and food, and they generally are healthy, but they still shoot their drugs.

"Hell," she laughed, "I was a *vegetarian* heroin addict. It's not like I didn't like my life or that I was trying to kill myself; it's just that I liked doing drugs and that was how I coped. I mean, I *still* like the idea of shooting dope; but I just realize that I can't do it and stay alive!"

And Lela clearly wants to stay alive and is working very hard toward that goal.

Narcotics Anonymous (NA) was very important to Lela in her early sobriety, but eventually she returned to drugs. "I was burned out. New York is a hard city to live in, and I realized that if I didn't go back to Portland, Maine, where I'm from, I'd never make it. So, I came back to Portland in June of 1985.

"And the first thing I did when I got back to Portland was shoot drugs, and that's when I tried to get in treatment. My life was pretty miserable, and I made a commitment to go to NA for one year. And they told me, 'If you don't like it after a year, we'll gladly refund your misery,'" she chuckled.

"In September of '85, I went and got tested for HIV. I was getting into a relationship with another woman. I got tested at a gay clinic, and not many women had used that clinic. The woman asked me a lot of questions, and I wasn't very honest. IV drug use was the only possible exposure route that I admitted to. Even today, if people ask me how I got exposed, I tend to say, 'It's not how I got here, it's what I'm gonna do while I'm here.'"

Her first antibody test was negative, but the counselor suggested that she be retested in six months. "I took this to mean that I was safe—that I was in the clear—and I put it out of my mind," Lela explained. "I wasn't told to change my habits; I figured I had nothing to worry about since the test was negative and I was four months clean at this time. I didn't get tested again in six months. Actually, I just forgot about it.

"In the spring of '86, I started having vaginal yeast infections that wouldn't clear up. Nothing worked. I was seeing a woman doc who knew my drug history, but I told her I had tested negative so she wasn't worried about AIDS. She was real calm about it."

But Lela's health problems continued to get worse. "I started developing respiratory illnesses, which I'd never had before. I was on antibiotics the whole time during April, May, and June, but the bronchitis didn't clear up. Then I got thrush in my mouth. Then the respiratory infection got really bad and my doctor suggested I get tested again. I did and it turned out I was HIV positive, and so they started to think that the things I was having were attributable to HIV."

Still, the diagnosis of ARC was never mentioned in '86, despite the fact that Lela's unusual health problems continued to progress. "Definitely something was wrong, but none of the doctors could figure out what. But in February of '87, I was diagnosed with presumptive PCP. I couldn't breathe. I was in total isolation. Everyone was masked and gowned and double-gloved. It was just hideous. They wouldn't let me use the bathtub!

"It was at this time that most people found out I was sick. Everyone thought I was going to die. They never actually cultured PCP, but they started me on Bactrim and I responded very well, and in April of '87 I began going to the hospital that handles all the AIDS cases.

"During the summer of '87, they weren't telling me I had ARC, but they were writing it in my chart. In September of '87 I got an official ARC diagnosis. I was profoundly symptomatic, and I'd been in the hospital every four months since this began. I'd had quite a lot of hospitalization for my lungs. I felt pretty overwhelmed and I hid a lot, and I didn't really talk a lot about it, but everyone knew. So I was 'out,' though I didn't have much choice."

At this crucial juncture in her life, Lela discovered the National Association of People with AIDS. Because NAPWA was eager to include more women with AIDS, Lela was sent an airline ticket to permit her to attend a national convention of People with AIDS taking place in Dallas, Texas.

"Meeting the women there and meeting you and other long-term survivors very profoundly changed my outlook," Lela recalled. "All of a sudden, I heard things I'd never thought of before—I'd never heard before. And instead of scaring me, it *empowered* me. Hearing that I didn't necessarily have to die was important. When I got my official ARC diagnosis, I thought, 'I'm going to die in a year!' Nobody said it to me explicitly, but they'd say things like, 'Do the things you want to do now while you still have your health.' Let's just say I'd picked up the message that the end was near, and by this time, I'd also begun to experience the death of friends."

Lela's previous extensive history of political involvement in the feminist, antinuclear, and Central American movements enabled her to quickly grasp the importance of PWA self-empowerment. She jumped in with both feet. "In October, I participated in the National March on Washington for Lesbian and Gay Rights. But in Washington, I started having seizures for the first time. And that really flipped me out! When I got home from the march, my neurological problems progressed. They said it was time to start AZT. Almost as an afterthought, I realized that the seizures and having to start AZT meant that I had progressed to AIDS."

For Lela, as for so many others, getting an official AIDS diagnosis was almost a relief. "Finally, we could start pinning something down. Before, I felt like I was a trivial woman with all sorts of minor ailments and that all I needed was to get my head in a better place in order to heal. I felt really insane, because even though I was doing all these drugs, I wasn't getting well and I didn't understand why."

One important difference for Lela after the NAPWA conference in Dallas was that she has insisted on receiving medication to prevent PCP whenever her T-cell count dips low. She believes that prophylaxis is a major reason why she's still here, although other respiratory problems have persisted despite the Bactrim. Periodically she has to have fluid drained from her lungs. "My weakest link is my lungs. They can never figure out what's going on. Sometimes they think it's viral or bacterial or fungal, but they never seem able to figure out exactly what it is. In May of '88, I had a very bad bout of pneumonia where I was in the hospital for eight weeks. Even though they never isolated PCP, they say it was PCP because I had infiltrates, bad oxygen levels, and everything."

Lela began AZT in October 1987, when she got her official AIDS diagnosis. Although she initially felt better on AZT—"it seemed to hold things at bay"—after nine months, doctors decided she should stop. "I take massive doses of anti-seizure medication and that works, for the most part. And I take two Bactrim tablets a day to prevent pneumonia. And two weeks out of every month, I take acyclovir to prevent herpes outbreaks. I find my herpes is very much hormonally related. I was on *so* many drugs that the doctors suggested I stop AZT because they didn't know what the possible drug interactions might be.

"I took AZT because I was afraid I was going to die and this was the drug that was supposed to keep me from dying. I went off AZT when I was hospitalized for presumptive PCP in the summer of '88.

"I started doing egg lipids in November of '87, just after starting AZT. I went off lipids in September of '88. At first, my T-cell counts went up, but no one knew whether it was lipids or AZT or both. Initially I thought lipids were really great, but now, in retrospect, I'm not too sure what to think. The best benefit I could see was that it tamed the herpes virus; my outbreaks were fewer and farther between. I have a couple of friends who started doing lipids at the same time as me and who are not sick and have maintained T-helper counts above 500. They had also tried AZT but quit because of the side effects. These two friends still really believe in lipids. I often think of doing them again, simply because they tame herpes."

Lela has explored other nontraditional approaches to healing. "Chiropractic, which helps me with my neuropathy and the very debilitating headaches I have sometimes; massage; macrobiotics; vitamins. I've run a whole gamut. I haven't done acupuncture. I listened to Louise Hay at first, but I think she's a capitalist pig and I don't want to support her at all. I just don't like her approach anymore. I have found people like Steve Levine and Elisabeth Kübler-Ross helpful, but again I wonder what they're doing with the money they get.

"I have found believing in some sort of higher power very helpful," Lela said. "And I do it only because it makes me feel good, not because I know that there's a Goddess or anything, but when I think there's no Goddess or no purpose to it all, then I feel hopeless. So it's just easier for me to believe that there's something out there.

"I've always been some strange quasi pagan. I was raised Lutheran and I needed something different. I have been much more into Native American spirituality. I've always had some strange quest to understand the spiritual side of life, but it wasn't until I got clean and sober that I began searching for that. I'm a born-again pagan," she joked. "I don't know. It just makes it easier on my psyche if I think that something exists out there."

Lela feels an obligation to help others who are newly diagnosed change their attitudes. She volunteers for an AIDS hotline and gives hope to countless frightened people. She also does AIDS education among IV drug users.

"Initially, I found support groups helpful. But now, I find two things happen in support groups. One my friend Pat and I call the 'Church of the Happy Face'—people who are HIV positive but not ill or newly diagnosed and into Louise Hay. I get really tired of listening to people talk about having the 'right attitude' or keeping a 'good attitude'—meaning that somehow those who have already died didn't do it right. It's like, get *real!* AIDS is no picnic! Or if they're not Church of the Happy Face, they're 'Poor me, poor me.' I hate people sitting around whining, 'Oh, I've got AIDS! Why me, why me?' And I kind of look around and say, 'Come on, *girl!* You had to *work* to get this disease. It's not like it tapped you on the shoulder one day while you were standing in line at the grocery store.' Yeah, it's traumatic, but let's go on with it.

"Pat and I started a women's support group. It's hard for me. I'm far enough into this illness that who I am frightens new people who come in, and so I tend to help *them*, rather than say what *I* really need. It's my service work. I do it so that other women won't be as alone as I was when this whole thing started. I don't do it because it gives me a lot of strength.

"Pat and I hold each other up. We both laugh before we cry, so we're good for each other. She was the first woman I met after my diagnosis. I can't imagine how things would be without her. I've also gotten a lot of support from gay friends who've since died of AIDS.

I also draw my inspiration from black literature, feminism, pagan spirituality. My spirituality is like the Cuisinart of Life—a little bit here, a little bit there, whatever makes me feel good at the time. But underlying it all is the Goddess, and earth-based/Native American religion."

Lela was in a relationship with a woman when she had ARC and through the period shortly after her AIDS diagnosis. "I come from a real dysfunctional family and so I've never felt worthy of love. I think I did everything I could to push the person away, and she said, 'I'm not leaving you.' That was amazing. Early on we were able to work together and she did a great deal of advocacy for me when I wasn't able to do it for myself. My lover was instrumental in helping me fight when I had given up.

"More than support groups, I have relied on my lover and my friends to help me get through the hard part. For me, AIDS is painful and hard. Day to day to day, there's never a moment that I don't have something happening."

I asked Lela why she broke up with the woman who had seen her through such hard times. She explained, "Trying to have a relationship in the world today—no matter who you are—is crazy enough. But then throw AIDS in on top of it all and you've got a mess. We lost friends both individually and together and it ended up that we relied on each other a lot—especially me on her. I've had times where I have been very sick. I've been paranoid. I've been in phases where intimacy—holding and touching and loving—were impossible. She was literally my lifeline—my link to doctors and the world. But it wasn't right that she had to live my life and her own.

"I also think that as my health has stabilized, I've needed to do and make my own decisions and bear the weight those decisions may bring. It's complex to explain, really. I think the bottom line is that I don't know how to love or be loved, and this has only been compounded by AIDS. I'm really grateful to have had the women who've been in my life. I don't think it's an understatement to say that if my lover hadn't been such a part of my life, I might not be here today. Her life seems to be taking off in new directions. I think she's happy not to be dragging me around the hospital rat track anymore," she laughed. And then she paused thoughtfully and said, "I love her very, very much.

"I might add, though, that I've all but given up hope of having another woman lover. These days, I am considered a great friend, but not dating material. I think it's quite clearly related to lesbian safe sex and the fact that few women want to, or are, doing it. Oh well. . . ." she sighed philosophically.

I asked her about her family's reaction to her diagnosis. "My family is a long way away, and they don't know how to deal with it. My mother takes this as her personal tragedy, and I just say, 'Give it up! This is *my* drama.' She relates to me like I'm dead and this is the worst thing that ever happened to *her*. I'm close to my sister, but that's about it."

I asked Lela why she thought she was still here, so far beyond all the dire predictions. "Because I'm too ornery to die," she stated matter-of-factly. "I'm planning a survival party for the end of October, just to say 'Fuck you' to the establishment. You know? 'I lived! Fuck you, fuck you! To spite you, I lived!' I've been an exception to the rules my whole life, and most of the time, I feel that if someone's gonna make it through this, it will be *me!* Why have I lived so long? I've changed *everything* in my life; I'm clean and sober. If I wasn't, I'd probably be dead by now, and I learned how to cope through NA. I'm no Big Book–thumper and I don't have the 'perfect' program; but I've got some new concepts to deal with old problems."

I asked Lela what advice she would give to a woman who had just been diagnosed with AIDS. "Be good to yourself. And I would give her my number and say, 'Anytime you need to call to talk, call me.' And I would encourage her to get into a support group—not to try to go through AIDS alone. I don't know anyone who is doing it alone and making it. And I'd tell her that knowledge is a tool of power. If you're unhappy with your doctor, find a different one."

Unlike other long-term survivors, Lela doesn't have any special relationship with her health care providers. "I'm pretty soured by the whole experience of medical doctors and the system. I don't have a doctor right now. I don't want to follow the traditional medical model. I want to work on treating separate viral infections that I have, rather than saying, 'Oh, it's all HIV and so there's nothing that can be done.' And most doctors aren't willing to do that. And we have about ten doctors who are dealing with 80 percent of the state's AIDS caseload. So, it's very hard to find doctors that aren't either burned out or afraid.

"I think I'm going to probably die of AIDS," she sighed. "But that doesn't bother me as much anymore. I'm sad about it sometimes, in the quiet times. But mostly I try not to think about it, and after all, everybody's got to die of something. I used to be afraid of death, but I'm not so much anymore because I've sat with so many friends who died, some in great struggle, but some very resolved and peacefully—that is, if dying can ever be considered peaceful."

Lela spoke out bitterly about some of the responses she has experienced as a long-term-surviving woman. "My case has gone up and down so much! When I'm well, I can be very well; and when I'm sick, I can be very sick. And people say, 'Well, maybe you don't *have* AIDS' or 'You look good'—because my cheeks are rosy with fever. But I really don't care whether I have AIDS or not anymore; I have an illness. This is it and I don't care what people say. I don't need to call it anything; it's just something that I need to live and deal with."

In such trying moments, Lela draws strength from several long-term survivors she knows. "My friend Dean's lived for five years. He's beat lymphoma and everything. So I say to myself, 'Well, I've only had full-blown AIDS for about two years, so that means I've got three more years,' or 'Michael's had AIDS for seven years, so that means I've got *five* more years.' I do that a lot and that gives me strength.

I know that I can be alive as long as you've been alive," she told me. "As long as I know there are other people out there who have done it, I can say, 'Well, they did it, so I can.' I know it's no guarantee, but those sorts of things are important for me."

"EMILIO"

"Fight with all your might."

▨▨▨ "Emilio" (not his real name) is a Latino gay man who answered my ad in the PWA *Newsline*. I met him for lunch *al fresco* in downtown Manhattan. He took me to a small, packed take-out restaurant that served unusually delicious food at a reasonable price.

When our interview took place in October 1987, Emilio was a thirty-nine-year-old, handsome, immaculately dressed, articulate gay man. He had moved to New York in 1970 from Puerto Rico. As he described how he came to be diagnosed, I learned how subtle racism can be.

"I was biopsied and diagnosed with KS in March of '84, but as early as November of '83 I had noticed lesions. The only thing is, I didn't recognize them as KS because the Gay Men's Health Crisis and all the gay papers said KS spots were purple; but mine were brown, so I thought they were moles."

I suddenly realized that KS is only purple or reddish if you're Caucasian; if you are black or brown-skinned, the lesions will probably not be pink. I wondered how many other people of color have ignored strange lesions because white gay-boy AIDS organizations have been telling everyone that KS lesions are purple or pink.

Actually, he said, he was glad to have had a couple of months of not having to deal with the trauma of an AIDS diagnosis.

Emilio struck me as spunky, optimistic, and good-natured. I asked him how finally being told that he had AIDS had affected him.

"Well, I went through a whole period of 'Oh, my God!' They were saying about how everyone dies. . . ." His voice trailed off in sadness. "But by about December of '84, I realized that I was still feeling very well. So I tried to be positive. I decided that it was not really going to beat me, and I figured there had to be some degree of survival, so why not me? And

I had tried also to inspire the same feeling in some friends of mine. I think fear has an awful lot to do with how we handle this sickness."

I asked Emilio if he had set out to be a survivor.

"No," he explained. "In the beginning I figured I only had eighteen months to live, like they usually quote. But when the eighteen months were up, I said, 'Well, here I am.' I was feeling no worse. I had more spots, but that was about it. Then two more years went by.

"It really gives me the creeps when I read the newspapers or watch TV," he said angrily. "Everything about AIDS is fatal, lethal, you know? No one is positive. That's why I'm doing this interview, because I think it's important for people who are recently diagnosed to find out that some of us are hanging in there. It's very disheartening that you never read about people who are really living with AIDS.

"You know," he continued, "people were saying things about being promiscuous, and I felt that that was really such a heavy trip to put on oneself. I hadn't done harm to anybody." Emilio admitted that he had "partied hard," which for him meant moderate use of recreational drugs and hundreds of sexual partners. But he angrily rejected the suggestion that his life-style had anything to do with his illness. He had concluded that AIDS was the result of something sinister.

"I have a heavy conviction that AIDS was not out of Mother Nature. I think it was something that was planted," he said forcefully. "I don't want to sound neurotic or paranoid, but I read a lot of things, and it seems like if they were going to try something like a virus, why not try it out on groups who are outcasts? But I figure the whole thing got a little bit out of hand."

Emilio was very well informed about his treatment options: "I'm currently taking dapsone to prevent PCP, and I'm taking naltrexone. I'm taking vitamins and drinking aloe vera juice, which I get in health food stores. I try to eat better."

But unlike other vitamin-popping holistic boosters, Emilio expressed a strong belief in the therapeutic value of alcohol. "I drink it every day—like a tonic," he said, laughing. "In fact, I haven't really changed my drinking habits at all. I drink like a fish! Every day—I mean, at night, not during the daytime. Usually vodka. I figure it has preserved all those people in Russia, so maybe it will do the same for me!"

Emilio has remained open minded about alternative approaches to AIDS. "To tell you the truth, if I was not working, I might have tried different approaches than I have." He said that his busy schedule and financial limitations prevented him from exploring massage, bodywork, and other therapies popular among PWAs. "But I do believe in alternative approaches to healing. For example, right now I'm carrying a crystal." He proudly produced a beautiful, bright rock.

Emilio, who works in a people-intensive, educational job, is selective about who he tells about his diagnosis. "My boss knows, but none of the other workers know. Fortunately I haven't had any lesions on my face, so I'm able to control who knows.

"Most of my family still lives in Puerto Rico, although I've managed to remain close to them. I have two brothers. One of them knows because he's a doctor; but my father doesn't know. Unless it was a question of really needing to, I will try not to inform him."

Emilio's mother died of cancer just prior to his diagnosis. He suspects that she knew he had AIDS: "On her deathbed, she kept asking me: 'Did you take care of those moles?' Because she had moles that turned out to be cancerous, she had a special concern for mine."

Emilio made it clear that he drew great strength from the love and support of his family and a few close friends. I asked him if he had also drawn strength from other PWAs or from other long-term survivors.

"Well, to tell you truly," he said, "I have attended some therapy groups, and I found them to be disappointing. I didn't find the feeling of positiveness that I was looking for. In the beginning, I figured I needed to be with people. After trying a support group, I realized it wasn't for me. But I try to connect with other PWAs now and then to see how things are going.

"I know a few other people with AIDS, but not many who've had the same positive attitude that I have. Sometimes I think it's fear that makes people really go down. I have a friend who is living in Bailey House, and he has a defeated attitude. He has always thought that nothing is going to change his AIDS verdict. He's sure he's gonna die. I say, 'Gosh, if there's 90 percent then there's also 10 percent, and so let me be part of that 10 percent!' Maybe I'm kidding myself, but I figured I'd just dust myself off and start all over again," he said cheerfully.

I couldn't imagine that someone so vivacious and handsome didn't have a lover, but Emilio described himself as "currently single, but definitely looking. I'm a romantic at heart." He said that his diagnosis had complicated his search for a lover. "I'm looking, but it's difficult. I figure the best way is to find somebody in the same boat. I've dated other PWAs, but so far, no luck. I sometimes think people are afraid to be committed, even if it's two PWAs who are in the same boat. I guess they fear that maybe one of them is going to go sooner.

"I had a crush on a friend of mine who also has AIDS. . . . Oh *God*, did I have a crush on him. I visited him when he was in the hospital. He said: 'Look at you . . . how good you look—brimming with health.' It is not easy being a survivor; sometimes I feel guilty. But I do have a few prospects." He winked.

"I've had no luck dating people who don't have AIDS. There have been times when I'd tell someone that I have AIDS and they'd run away. They say they're glad I'm being honest, but then they always say good-bye!"

Emilio has no intention of sitting idle while he's waiting to meet the love of his life. In addition to finding fulfillment in his job, his family, and friends, he has discovered that he loves to travel.

"Initially, my doctor said it was a good idea for me to take a break from the stress. I took a sick leave from my job and got full pay because it had been authorized by my doctor. I really needed the rest, and it did me a lot of good. Now I take advantage of opportunities that come my way.

"When I went to Brazil in 1984, I figured that that was going to be my last trip. Then, lo and behold, I was still here in '85. And I was still here in '86. And this is '87, and I'm still here. To celebrate, I went to India. India was very interesting and relaxing," he said.

Besides a desire to travel to more exotic places, Emilio has other dreams that he believes help keep him alive. "I have many goals. I'd like to be in the fashion world. I like to design clothes. And one of the things I've said is if I'm ever free of AIDS—if I ever go into remission—I'm going to see if I can get into fashion. It's never too late, you know.

"Also, I have lost a lot of good friends. Very close friends. And I had somehow said to myself that I have to at least survive so that their deaths were not in vain. I know that sounds a little bit crazy, but I really feel that if there had been some more positive things in the past, people would have been able to have lived longer.

"I guess it's my karma to survive," he said philosophically. "I have friends who were diagnosed after me who are already gone! Maybe it's God's design that I'm supposed to still be here. I don't know. Maybe I'm supposed to be an example, and eventually to even go public. Anyway, I'm still alive and still fighting."

I asked him if his doctor had ever told him he was doomed.

"Nope," he answered. "I have a very good doctor. He is *fantastic*. But other people in the medical field have told me that they don't believe that anyone can survive AIDS. But in every study I have been in, I become like a mascot because of my positive attitude and the fact that I've survived so long," he said proudly.

Emilio thinks his doctor's approach to treatments plays an important role in his long-term survival.

"My doctor is very cautious about what treatments he recommends for me. For example, even though I feel a little bit self-conscious about my spots (I call myself 'the leopard'), he says no chemotherapy unless it's absolutely necessary. And I have followed his judgment. To tell you the truth," he laughed, "I sometimes forget about my doctors' appointments because I feel so well."

I asked him if there was anything else besides good doctoring and a positive attitude that he felt played a major role in his long-term survival.

"I became a Buddhist in 1972. I'm not as religious as I was at first, but something has been telling me that I really should get more heavily into it. I should be a little more disciplined."

Emilio's Buddhism has helped him view death as nothing more than a natural part of the life cycle. "The moment that you're born, your chances of dying are right there," he explained. "It all just depends on what your time is set up for. I think that in some cases, due to this health crisis, people's time is a little bit ahead of schedule.

"But still," he said, "you can be crossing the street and die." Laughing, he recalled a tense moment that occurred during a recent flight to Puerto Rico. "We had a lot of turbulence and I said, 'Ain't no way that this plane is gonna crash, because I cannot be diagnosed with AIDS and then die in a plane crash. I mean, that is too much punishment!' "

We had finished our lunch and Emilio said he had to get back to work. I asked him a final question: "What advice would you give to somebody who came to you and said, 'I was just diagnosed 15 minutes ago. Tell me what you've learned from your experience. What should a PWA do?' "

He thought for a moment and then said: "Fight with all your might and try to beat the odds. I am thoroughly convinced that the basic thing you need to conquer this is a positive attitude. True, if you're having a rash or if you're experiencing other health problems, you sometimes wonder. But the mind is very strong. So having a positive attitude would be my recommendation. And get all the information that you can get."

I told him he seemed really well adjusted to his diagnosis. I asked him if he had always been so cheerful and positive.

"You know, it's a funny thing," he answered. "When I was younger, I used to have this ugly-duckling feeling. It was just lack of confidence. I worked very hard to come out of the closet and like myself. I even learned to enjoy looking at myself in the mirror—to feel good about myself. And then suddenly I'm diagnosed with AIDS. And so I said, I can't have come such a long way, baby, only to be turned back to point zero by this disease! I intend to make my life work. I intend to be a survivor!

"Besides," he confided, "I'm dying to find out if I'm right about AIDS being a government conspiracy. Then I'll be able to say, 'See! I told you so!' Obviously, I have to be *alive* in order to say that," he laughed.

"ROBERTO"

"I'm alive because I chose to be alive."

▨▨▨ When my friends in the holistic AIDS community learned I was profiling long-term survivors, they were eager for me to meet and interview "Roberto" (not his real name).

At the time of our interview in October 1987, Roberto had survived KS for over five years. He is one of the most famous AIDS success stories in holistic/AIDS circles, in particular among those committed to Michio Kushi and macrobiotics.

Although we travel in similar AIDS circles, I hadn't met Roberto before. I was, frankly, worried that he would have that EST-ian, glassy-eyed automaton quality that many of those committed to certain healing philosophies exhibit. But when I met him in his lovely Chelsea apartment, I found a warm, articulate survivor who literally glowed with health. Over delicious (and no doubt healthful) tea, we two PWAs dished the survival dirt.

"I was never officially diagnosed by the medical profession as having AIDS. In 1982, I went to one of the real cancer mills, which shall remain nameless. They biopsied one of my lesions and they said it was KS. I also had swollen lymph nodes in my groin, under my jaw, and under my arms. The right side of my body was withering; I was losing control over the movement in my right hand and right leg. And there was an overall immune system deterioration going on. At the time, nobody knew what it was."

Roberto explained that prior to AIDS, the doctors at this "cancer mill" were familiar with KS as a disease that occurred primarily in Italians and Jews over sixty. Roberto had been married for twenty years and had two children; but as a bisexual who had been very sexually active after his divorce, Roberto definitely had a history of AIDS risk behavior. "Because

I was forty-eight in 1982, and because I am Italian," Roberto explained, "the cancer mill doctors preferred to believe I only had 'regular' KS. They told me I was the youngest case of 'regular' KS that they had ever seen!

"Although they never officially said that I might have AIDS, they were apparently suspicious," he said. "After I had the lesion removed and biopsied, I was sent for extensive blood testing. They wanted to do all the 'oscopies'—the bronchoscopies, the colonoscopy, endoscopy, whatever. And they also wanted to remove one of my lymph nodes and test it for cancer."

Deciding whether to allow invasive diagnostic procedures proved to be a turning point for Roberto. "I was very fortunate. I had a really strong spirit guide and teacher in my life for years—Maxine—and she said to me, 'Remove your lymph nodes?! That's one of your sentinels against illness.' I decided that allowing them to remove my lymph node would only further impair my immune system. So I chose not to do that.

"A big, giant wall went up. I said, 'Cease and desist. I no longer want to play in your arena.' And I stepped away from modern medicine. This was really early in '82. And then I started searching for another way."

Roberto has never regretted his decision to eschew Western medicine, with all its high-tech poking and prodding and potent chemotherapeutic agents. Offered interferon therapy for his KS, he turned it down. He strongly suspected that his KS was AIDS related and he decided to search for "another way" to heal himself.

His search led him to investigate the role of diet in healing. "A friend sent me a book about a healing diet which recommended eating lots of fruit, and no meats except chicken occasionally. And no dairy," he recalled. "It seemed very interesting to me. Actually, I refused to read the section on cancer. That's what a shock it was to me at that point. I mean, I was devastated by the whole thing."

But after adapting this diet to include "things like honey, vanilla, carob ice cream—you know, 'healthy' ice cream," he joked, "a year later things were not getting better. In fact, things were continually deteriorating. And I asked, 'Where is the next clue going to come from?' I figured I'd trust the universe and see what happened. I was also exercising and I was taking control of my life."

At a party one night, another woman friend suggested that Roberto buy Michio Kushi's book on macrobiotics. Roberto sensed that this was the clue he'd been waiting for.

"I went to the bookstore and found Michio's book. At that point I had $15 to my name, and the book was reduced from $15.95 to $11—which is never, *ever* done. So there was really a very strong guiding hand.

"In 1983, while reading Kushi's book, I kept on saying to myself 'No. No, no.' Every now and then I'd find my head bobbing up and down saying 'Maybe . . . Well, yeah. . . .' And then I found my head *only* going up and down. Suddenly something in me went 'click' and I saw that if you applied the basic principles of macrobiotics to your life, it *had* to work. I just saw the clarity of it all. And I took that leap of faith and embraced macrobiotics. I've been macrobiotic ever since."

Eventually, Roberto joined a group called Wipe Out AIDS (WOA), which was one of the first New York City groups of "holistic heretics" to explore alternative approaches to dealing with AIDS.

Michio Kushi is a somewhat controversial figure. His detractors make much of the fact that he smokes tobacco and has been known to enjoy an alcoholic beverage now and then. But Kushi is widely respected in holistic circles for his ability to articulate the principles behind macrobiotics. And unlike some holistic practitioners, who have kept their distance from AIDS, Kushi has been personally involved in examining the potential of macrobiotics as an AIDS therapy. Roberto works closely with Michio Kushi and his wife, Avelino.

"I put the question of my diagnosis very directly to Mr. Kushi, because I wanted it clarified in my own mind," Roberto told me. "He classified me from his point of view as 'pre-AIDS.' "

Although some of his original KS lesions are fading, Roberto has continued to develop new ones. "But only on my legs," he points out. Roberto has remained committed to macrobiotics and believes that his new lesions are "basically carbonized meat and sugar that are buried very deeply in my body which are now coming to the surface. Perhaps to most people it seems like I'm fooling myself into believing that, but that's what I think it is. And when I presented my lesions to Michio, he looked at them and asked, 'What do *you* think they are?' I told him my theory and he said, 'You're right.' The way I look at it, I would rather they came to the surface than were buried in my body."

Roberto said he felt that besides helping some of his lesions fade, his commitment to macrobiotics was having other beneficial effects. "I have renewed energy, an energy that I never before experienced in my life. I have an energy which comes directly from the foods I eat instead of coming from all the other things I used to use to create the emotional reactions. Primarily drugs," he admitted frankly. "I did drugs for many, many years. At the time, it seemed like there was no other way to live."

Roberto's sex and drug use history was similar to that of most gay men with AIDS. "I would smoke about an ounce of grass a week. On difficult days, I would take an up, in the form of a small diet pill—which incidently," he spat contemptuously, "had been prescribed by my *doctor*. I mean, we all manage to get what we want out of our lives, don't we?

"I also used to take penicillin prophylactically after sex. So I was taking antibiotics daily, since I didn't consider it a normal day if I didn't have sex at least once or twice." Roberto used other recreational drugs as well. His favorite was Quaaludes.

Like most PWAS, Roberto went through an initial "Why me?" period, which led him to do a painful emotional housecleaning. "When I was diagnosed in '82, I went into shock. I had daily crying bouts, wondering what I had done—'Why me?' I was a *total* victim. And when I finally stopped crying long enough to look at what I was doing, I decided that the first thing I had to do was to give up drugs. I worried, 'But I'll be socially ostracized. I won't have any *friends* left.'

"And then I started analyzing all of my friends and how many of them did drugs, and I realized very clearly that none of my real friends did drugs. In fact, I was always trying to convince *them* to do drugs," he recalled.

Many people have commented on the numbers of long-term survivors who speak like they're members of an Alcoholics Anonymous twelve-step program. Although many people with AIDS have used AA and NA for their alcohol and drug addictions, many long-term survivors discovered on their own the value of applying the twelve-step principles to their struggle to survive AIDS.

"I went cold turkey off drugs and I started out one day at a time," Roberto said. "I didn't know 'one day at a time' was an AA principle, 'cause I'd never been to any of those groups."

Taking AIDS one day at a time, Roberto reached June 21, 1982—his birthday—and realized that it had been a long time since he'd done marijuana. At this crucial turning point, fate again seemed to intervene. He discovered some marijuana hidden in his medicine cabinet and, in a moment of weakness, decided to light up.

"I took out one joint, went into the bedroom, lit it and discovered I had to take a leak. So I went back into the bathroom with the joint in my mouth, drawing on it, but the joint hadn't actually caught fire. Then, when I went to the john to urinate, it fell in the john. And I said to myself, 'The universe is telling you something.' "

He decided to take a hint and flushed the remaining pot down the toilet. "Now, whenever June 21 rolls around, I count it off as being another year; and it's been over five years now. I haven't even had aspirin. No drugs."

Roberto also gave up sex cold turkey. "I didn't think I could exist without sex. But I wasn't even interested in masturbating at that point.

It was like the ovens were turned off. I really felt that I had the plague, and as a responsible person, I would not risk passing it on to anyone else. Besides, explaining it all to a potential sex partner would have been just too complicated." Eventually, however, Roberto began to have safer sex with others.

"After being macrobiotic for five years, all my blood work is normal," he told me proudly. "It's been normal for the longest time. I mean, I don't even think of myself as having. . . ." He didn't finish his sentence, as if saying the word "AIDS" might jinx his success. "Only when I look around at others am I reminded that there's a possibility that there's something there," he said.

After his health stabilized, Roberto experienced the healing power of love. "I had an affair last year that I really thought was the all-time, ultimate affair. I met someone who had many of the same interests I had in life. And I thought it was really perfect. And then suddenly it just all fell apart. It was really shocking to me. I was angry and bitter and upset, but now I realize that it taught me that love was something that could occur in my life again—that the possibility is always there. You have to be open to it when it comes and however it turns out, it turns out. And I would not want to have denied myself the experience of that relationship. It's fun to be able to cuddle with somebody and kiss someone and sleep with them."

I asked Roberto how he deals with people who are not pursuing a macrobiotic approach. "It's much easier for somebody who is macrobiotic to be with others who are macrobiotic, because then, that whole confrontation about your-food-versus-my-food doesn't have to take place. It's not that I don't have friends who aren't macrobiotic, but I find it much easier to be around others who are.

"In the beginning it was weird. I used to feel that if someone couldn't be convinced to become macrobiotic, it would really stand in the way of my *own* recovery. I had to learn to separate myself from that—to leave people their freedom to make their own choices.

"I think a lot of times what happened was that people who really didn't have clear insights as to what macrobiotics really means became proselytizers—instead of just being people who are representative of what the principles are. I used to be that way. But now I don't proselytize. If somebody wants information about macrobiotics, I'm willing to give it to them. But I don't preach."

Roberto also expressed frustration that many people mistakenly believe that macrobiotics is only about diet.

"It's not only about food," he explained. "Macrobiotics is about principles—the way you conduct your life. It's a philosophy about how to live in harmony. One of the most important principles of macrobiotics is 'Non fado,' " he explained. "It means 'Don't believe us.' "

I was intrigued. "Non fado" sounded like the Oriental version of the principle of radical doubt that has guided my own response to AIDS.

"The macrobiotic philosophy is presenting ideas; if those ideas fit into your life, if they intrigue you enough to want to study further, okay. And macrobiotics needn't conflict with any other beliefs—Catholicism, Buddhism, whatever. Macrobiotics is only in *addition* to.

"And you don't have to become Japanese to become macrobiotic!" he said, laughing. "There are always different ways of channeling energy, and macrobiotics is just part of a whole tapestry of our lives that can help create all the other options that are open to us."

I asked Roberto whether the fact that no one has ever officially said that he has AIDS had cushioned him from all the negative propaganda. "Yeah, but up until this June, I really considered myself as someone with AIDS. Even though I wasn't officially diagnosed as having AIDS by Michio Kushi or by modern medical professionals, I suddenly started realizing that if I was going to be used as an example of macrobiotics, in a *sub rosa* context, that I didn't want to be making statements about modern medicine or about macrobiotics which could be refuted by the medical profession. Because the burden of proving that macrobiotics is a good recovery tool falls on *macrobiotics*, it doesn't fall on Western medicine or the rest of the world. So I wanted to be very clear that Michio perceived me as having originally had AIDS. Because I didn't want to make false statements about macrobiotics as a healing tool for AIDS."

In fact, Roberto was a driving force behind a formal, scientific study of people with AIDS on macrobiotics. Researchers Eleanor Levy and John Beldekas of Boston University have studied a group of gay men with KS, recruited largely from the WOA support group. Initial results of the study were published in a major medical journal and found that all the men with KS who were macrobiotic were doing as well, if not better, than those pursuing other treatment approaches to their AIDS-related KS.

"I think that is an incredible finding," Roberto said proudly. "Michio says, 'Every day wake up and sing a happy song and just live your life like you're not ill.' "

I shifted uncomfortably in my seat. Kushi's quote seemed glib and simplistic. Sensing my discomfort, Roberto translated Kushi's advice into language that was more accessible to someone like me. "When you're really standing at the precipice of death, you have to make a decision about whether you're going to leap in or whether you're going to pull back and stay here," he said. "I consciously decided that I had more to do on this planet, and that I had to find a way to stay here.

"Actually, macrobiotics is not an easy thing for most people to do," Roberto admitted, "because most of us would rather continue leading our lives and take some medication so that we don't have to be actively involved in our recovery. And I think that's the biggest difference I see in people who choose macrobiotics. Instead of becoming victimized by their illness, people involved with macrobiotics are participating in their own recovery."

Roberto had an interesting theory about what he called "the big picture" of AIDS. "A year before I got KS, I was really looking for a way out. And I suddenly felt that death was really an option. To create within myself an illness that was *the* newest illness—a disease that I could die from—would be a way for society to condone my death without my having to throw myself off a building. But when I really got to the point where death was a possibility, I asked myself 'Do you really want to die or do you want to do something about this?' And I opted to do something about it."

In addition to macrobiotics, Roberto also finds strength and comfort in his Catholicism and in meditation. "When I meditate," he said, "my life really works. Interestingly, part of my self-destructive way of living my life is that I sometimes refuse to do something that's so obviously valuable to me. I think that's probably a very strong trait of a lot of homosexuals. If we find out that something works, we go 'Oh! That works? *Now* what are we going to do? Let's move on to the next thing.' " He laughed.

"I have also returned to my Roman Catholic heritage. I try to pray daily in a meditative state." Roberto carefully distinguished his Catholicism from the judgmental, harsh religion of many Catholics: "I have my own individual relationship with God that has nothing to do with the official church. I happen to like formalized structure. I like the drama and pageantry of the Roman Church. But at the same time, it's very sad for me to see what the Catholic Church is doing to gay people."

Roberto is strangely half-in and half-out of the AIDS closet. Many people within the macrobiotic community know of his diagnosis, but he's not willing to be completely public. "I'm very careful about what I say. I have never publicly claimed that I have been 'cured' or that I am 'recovered completely.' But you can't control what other people say. A lot of people interpret what I say in whatever way they need for themselves," he said.

"I'm alive," Roberto said passionately, "because I chose to be alive. I really want to discover what all the other things are that I'm here to do.

I've become a spokesperson for macrobiotics and AIDS. I really want to be a living manifestation of the principles working in somebody's life. I want to prove to people that macrobiotics is not just an abstraction. I think that when you get to the point where you're doing very well, you should put it back out there in the universe."

Roberto exudes a calm optimism. It's very clear that *he's* very clear about the direction he wants his life to take.

I asked him if he believed he was destined to die from AIDS.

"No," he answered emphatically. "I think my AIDS will just burn itself out."

I ended our interview with the same final question I had asked other survivors: What advice would he give to someone newly diagnosed?

"First thing I would say is, if you feel like crying, please cry. And if it goes on for three weeks, cry and let it all out and let yourself go beyond your level of being victimized by the illness. Then get on with your life. Then when you're ready to sit down and talk, let me hold you and we'll talk about it. And let me just share with you some books that you might want to read.

"There are options other than the ones seemingly available. Macrobiotics is only one option. You may decide to stand on your head and get well. I don't know what your choice will be, but it will be different from my choice, or somebody else's choice. And even if you choose to do what I've chosen to do, you may do it in your way, which would be different from the way I'd do it."

"HELMUT"

"Don't give up!"

⊠⊠⊠ "Helmut" (not his real name) is a survivor in two senses of the word: He has survived the death of his lover from AIDS and has himself survived AIDS-related Kaposi's sarcoma since 1982. Although he has been very active in the political fight against AIDS, he has chosen not to publicly identify himself as a PWA.

"Actually," he explained, "there are only two or three people who know that I have AIDS. I don't particularly want my friends to find out by reading it in an interview."

Helmut began dealing with AIDS long before the term "AIDS" even existed. His lover, "Sam" (also an alias), was one of the first in New York City to be diagnosed with GRID.

"Denial" is a bad word to most people. But Helmut's experience suggests that denial can have its uses.

Despite the appearance of KS lesions in 1982, it wasn't until the summer of '86 that Helmut's doctors finally used the word "AIDS" to refer to his condition.

"It wasn't until four years after my first lesion that the actual word 'AIDS' was spoken. Sam had died in January of '81. Within a year, I had developed this spot on my arm." As people with AIDS tend to do, Helmut rolled up his sleeve to show me his first "spot." In a uniquely eighties slice of gay life, we compared lesions.

"See this?" he said. "You can hardly see it. It's dissolved. But not the other lesions. I obviously have a very slowly progressing case of KS."

Friends supported his avoidance of the term "AIDS" and all its stigmas. "I didn't really even think about it. I even showed the lesion to people, and all of them laughed and said, 'Oh, come on! Not you. Not KS.' But I had seen people with lesions, so I knew what they looked like. But I clung to the fact that this first one didn't really look like most lesions."

Another factor that encouraged denial was that Helmut was used to developing "spots." "I'm one of those people who has moles; they run in my family. So growths on my body have been something that I grew up with. My brother, my mother, my father, and myself have always had them removed every once in a while."

In 1981, he showed his first lesion to one of the foremost AIDS experts, who had enrolled Helmut in a prospective study of AIDS. "Nothing was ever said," he recalled. As other lesions developed, Helmut kept showing them to this doctor. "He kept saying, 'Oh, isn't that funny . . . they disappear. Gee, I don't know what it is. . . .' And that was exactly what I wanted to hear. So, I figured 'Fine. There's no real problem here.' "

This curious song and dance went on for three years, sparing Helmut from having to deal with dire predictions that he ought to be dead.

But slowly, more lesions appeared. Still, neither the AIDS researcher, Helmut's dermatologist, nor his general practitioner ever said, "You have AIDS." "The word just did not come out of their mouths, maybe because there was really nothing else wrong with me. Oh, I have a little bit of thrush in my mouth once in a while. But other than that, I have had no energy loss, no weight loss."

I asked Helmut if he harbored any anger toward the doctors. Just the opposite, he said. "I sort of *eased* into my diagnosis. And even though nobody said it to me, I really knew it. 'Helmut,' I said to myself, 'you have AIDS.' But I liked it that nobody else said it. In the end, my doctors told me that the way I handled it was perfectly right."

Another reason why Helmut has survived so long may be that he avoided the violently aggressive, immunosuppressive chemotherapies that may have hastened the death of many of those diagnosed with AIDS in the early days. Like other survivors, he was very well-educated about the sad state of AIDS treatment research. "I read a lot and I have kept on top of everything since this started. I keep a running list of all the new drugs that come out, and somewhere along the line I ask my doctors about them."

But Helmut shares other survivors' generally skeptical attitude about potentially toxic experimental drugs. "I figure there must be something in my body dealing with this, since it's progressing as slowly as it is. So I don't want to take something like AZT and *kill* myself! So, I'm very, very careful."

But Helmut keeps an open mind about nontoxic, holistic approaches to AIDS. On the recommendation of one doctor, he tried egg lipids. "The only side effect," he amusingly noted, "was a resurgence of sexual desire.

"I'm also trying bee propolis. It's from Sweden and it's a natural substance that bees create. A beehive doesn't have bacteria in it, because bees create this gummy substance called propolis that keeps the hive sterile. You chew it like gum; it works as a natural antibiotic."

Helmut is an extremely handsome, sexy, cheery gay man with a gravelly voice suggestive of a male version of Lauren Bacall. When I interviewed him in October 1987, he said he was forty-three. He looked many years younger.

I asked him how AIDS had affected his sex life. "Most of my friends have died," he reported sadly. "My lover and I don't have a great deal of sex anymore. I mean, we can go months without having sex. I was a product of Flamingo," he said, referring to one of New York's first gay discos—some say it was the prototypical disco mythologized in Andrew Holleran's classic saga of the urban gay fast lane of the seventies, *Dancer from the Dance.* "But unlike others, I would only take drugs to go dancing. And never acid or mescaline; and never, never ethyl. Poppers, yes. And, oh, coke, grass, PCP, and some of those minor things."

He considered that his sex life was more moderate than most of the Flamingo crowd's. "Sure, I went to the baths; but my sexuality was basically with my lover."

When Sam died, Helmut grieved for a while before taking another lover. When that relationship broke up, Helmut met his current lover. "We had known each other for a long, long time and we used to spend the night dancing. He always used to ask me to go home with him and I always used to say, 'I'm still in the throes of dealing with the situation with my previous lover' and so I never went—not until I had broken up with that previous lover."

Helmut returned to the topic of why he has chosen not to tell most people that he has AIDS. "I don't see any reason why I need to tell more friends or my family. They have enough to deal with with everyone else who is sick or dying. And I just don't have problems with my diagnosis."

He paused to reconsider his last statement. "The only time that I get a little emotionally jarred is when I'm standing in front of the mirror brushing my teeth. I don't like looking at myself with these spots. But," he said, brightening, "there's nothing I can do about it. I'm one of those people who has a pretty 'up' attitude about things. I'm able to keep my energies pretty high, so I can get through all this without everybody needing to know."

Helmut got momentarily pensive. He explained, "For me, family comes first. And when I say 'family,' I don't necessarily mean my blood relatives. Out of a group of about twenty people who I was friends with on Fire

Island over the years, only three of us are left. Now, I put my energies into my lover and my mother and father. My family and I emigrated from Europe in 1952, so I have no other family to speak of, except a brother who I'm certainly not close to."

Helmut denied that fear of discrimination plays any role in his choosing not to be public as a PWA. "Being anonymous in this interview has nothing to do with fear of discrimination. This just isn't the way I want my friends to find out. I'm certainly not in the closet as a gay man; and as you know, I've been very active in AIDS work. I just want to make that clear.

"Frankly, politics is something that I could have done without all my life. I was into art, music, and so on. But I have become very political. And I find I enjoy working in gay and AIDS politics."

I asked him why he thought he had survived KS for so long. "Two reasons," he said. (He had clearly asked himself this question many times before.) "One reason is genetics. Both my mother and father are seventy-seven years old. My mother's mother just died about a month ago; she was ninety-nine. My father's father died at 103. I remember my great-grandmother, who died at 107."

Like several other long-term survivors, Helmut has a history of triumphing over adversity. "I had TB as a kid. In fact, I had all the major diseases, and I came through those. That was right after World War II, with all the food shortages and other hardships. I think that helped make my body strong, and that, coupled with my genes, must be factors in my surviving AIDS.

"Another factor is my attitude. I'm not prone to being negative or depressed. That doesn't mean I don't get that way sometimes, but usually it'll only last a day or two, and then I always manage to rally. So genes and attitude are the two things I credit for my survival."

Also, luck. "I feel really lucky, first of all, that I've survived this long, since I must have been one of the first people infected. I'm also lucky because I met several fellow long-term survivors. There was Phil Lanzarata, of course. And Bob. And Ray. I know a number of others who've had AIDS from the very beginning, like me."

I asked Helmut how he reacted to the gloom-and-doom media campaign. He laughed good-naturedly: "When I hear some newscaster say 'Everybody dies from AIDS,' I want to tap the TV set and raise my hand! I'm sure there are others out there like me and you who could use a little slap on the back, as if to say 'It's okay, there are others of us and. . . .' Who knows?" he mused. "Maybe we hold the key to survival for others. I don't understand why they haven't studied us more closely. For instance, why do I have slowly progressing KS?"

Helmut chose not to join a PWA support group. "I'd rather be on the caring end than be cared for," he explained. "I don't feel I need to be cared for, because there's nothing wrong right now that is getting in the way of leading a normal life."

What advice would he give to someone newly diagnosed who wants to enter the long-term-survival sweepstakes?

"Read *every* thing!" he exclaimed. "That way you'll feel you aren't helpless. Make lists of your options, including holistics. Be reasonable. I'm not a pill taker, but I will take them when they have to be taken. But if I can get around it, I will.

"And always, always have hope. You see, I definitely believe in an afterlife. I go to church from time to time, when it's empty, to pray. Because I want to be closer to God. I pray every night—talk to God in my own way. I have a running relationship with him," he joked.

"I'm more spiritual than religious. I also believe in karma and reincarnation. I have felt all my life that I died in a concentration camp in the Second World War and was reincarnated very quickly. I just feel that way. You're only the second person I've ever said that to," he confided, surprising us both.

He summarized his own survival philosophy very simply: "Don't give up!"

"EDDIE"

"It's not the quantity, it's the quality."

▨▨▨ It was a brutally cold day in late November 1987 when I schlepped up to Harlem with my bulky tape recorder to interview "Eddie" (not his real name), a very handsome, articulate, gay black man. I had been introduced to Eddie through a mutual friend who hadn't prepared me for *how* handsome he was.

Eddie was born and raised in New York City and, at the time of our interview, was thirty-three. Prior to his diagnosis, he worked as a video editor. He had quit his job and was now spending a lot of time volunteering at the Minority Task Force on AIDS. "If I'm going to do office work, I'd rather work with the Minority Task Force and help those people that are like myself, you know?" he said.

Eddie's apartment was huge, with a nice view, lots of light, very little furniture, and a roommate who was sleeping in a bedroom far away. I always feel uncomfortable whipping out all this sound equipment. But Eddie immediately put me at ease and began to tell his story.

"I was only diagnosed in December of '86. And I only came down with PCP." I was startled to hear him say "only PCP." But as I learned, his generally optimistic nature leads him to minimize bad things and emphasize good things.

"I had tested negative for HIV back in March of '86. So getting PCP was a complete surprise and I was in the hospital for five and a half weeks, on a respirator for a while. The only sign I had while I was getting PCP was that I started getting diarrhea. I thought it was part of the flu. I had been having sweats for a while before that, but I didn't really look at them as abnormal because the apartment was kind of hot, and I sleep with a blanket," he said.

"Actually I was walking around with pneumonia. The first time I went to the emergency room, they diagnosed me with the flu. They gave me Robitussin cough medicine and Tylenol and they said, 'Take this and you'll feel better in a few days; if you don't, come back.' I was back the next morning and it turned out to be PCP."

I asked Eddie if he was satisfied with his health care. "I go to Metropolitan Hospital Clinic," he explained, "because I was enrolled in a health maintenance program. I'm on public assistance—Medicaid and Social Security Disability. Now I go to the AZT-AIDS outpatient clinic at Metropolitan. It was one of the first hospitals to get involved with AZT.

"I started taking AZT at the end of February and I'm doing well. I also don't do exactly as they say, taking it every four hours. I take it when I'm *aware* of it. I'm doing fine on AZT. I've had no side effects. At least, I'm under control and I'm being watched and I see them taking my blood and my blood counts are all coming up and the doctors are really tripping out. I've heard people and their negativity toward AZT, and that's fine. Whatever pills I take, I don't know what the eventual outcome is going to be. So this is working, so fuck it. I mean, what have I really got to lose? Either way I could lose."

But I was disappointed to learn that he had not been put on any form of PCP prevention therapy. "Somebody mentioned something to me, but I kind of feel that I won't get PCP again, because when I came down with it the first time, I thought it was because I hadn't dressed properly, going out wet, which I don't do at all anymore. Like, I didn't go out yesterday because it was so cold. And when I do go out, I have on a turtleneck, a sweater, ski pants, a ski jacket, gloves, and a hat. Everybody stares at me going down in the elevator," he laughed. "It's like they want to say, 'Well, all you need is ski poles!' "

Eddie is aware of the treatment "underground," but it doesn't interest him. "I just didn't trip on trying other things. Actually, I've talked to a few people. My mother works with a couple of people that've come down with AIDS. And they run to Mexico, and they're doing this and doing that; doing everything! Everything that's out there, they're doing it. But it's weird to me when I see that. You don't know what the chemical reaction to all these things you're doing might be."

Eddie told me that he wasn't sure whether he'd gotten AIDS from his IV drug use or from his bisexual activity. He said he didn't really think much about it though. "I've shot up and I did share the needle. So maybe. But I don't worry about it really, because it's sexually transmitted and so everybody's at risk. It's just not important how I got it. And hey, I think there's more to AIDS than what they think there is. And AIDS isn't new. It might have something to do with syphilis. It's about life-styles that we're leading today, with drug abuse and the environment, with promiscuity and diseases. I mean, I've had syphilis and hepatitis."

But Eddie was adamant that he hadn't shot up drugs very frequently and also said that he hadn't been all that promiscuous. "I didn't do bathhouses or tearooms. I preferred having sex with people I was having a relationship with," he explained. "Actually, there was a period where I had a lot of sex, but basically, when I tripped sexually, it was with people I loved. I mean, if it's just physical, I'd rather be by myself. I get more being by myself and masturbating than I'd get with a stranger, you know?"

Actually, I told him, I *didn't* know. I had been a slut, like many urban gay men who came of age in the seventies. Back then, I always admired anyone who actually found intimacy sexy.

Eddie considers himself more gay than bisexual, although just before he came down with PCP, he had been planning to get married. "I wanted to marry a woman because I wanted to have children and she was somebody who knew my trip. We had a relationship already, and she wanted children too. She's thirty-two years old. Her clock is ticking down, and it was like, 'Well, fuck it, what do we have to lose? We're friends. It would be nice to establish a healthy sexual relationship, but if we don't, that's fine too.' We'd just work around it. Basically we'd become engaged. But we subsequently called it off after I was diagnosed. We're still friends, although I haven't seen her in a while."

Lowering his voice, Eddie confided to me that he was in love with the roommate who was asleep down the hall. "He's like my best friend, and it's weird. I've always had a deep affection for him, but nothing sexual has ever transpired. I've fallen in love with him, and I don't know if he knows. I'm trying to bring it out, but I'm afraid it will change the relationship, because I don't think he feels the same way. I know he *loves* me, but maybe he doesn't know how much. I've started psychotherapy because I've got to work this out before I go crazy," he laughed. "We've known each other since '82," Eddie said. "Since I got sick, he's been my biggest supporter."

Eddie doesn't like support groups. "I don't like listening to people who feel sorry for themselves. I know AIDS isn't an easy thing to take. I mean, it kind of tripped me. But I knew I was at risk! AIDS is out here. So fine; now I have it. And now I do what they tell me to do to get better, you know—things that I know might help make me better. Actually I get freaked out when I see people who are too sick.

"With AIDS, you get to see who your friends are, you know? Most of my friends are supportive, and I don't even worry about those who aren't.

I'm my own best friend. So that's all that really matters. Of course, you do need a little encouragement on the side.

"My family is basically supportive," he continued. "I grew up in a single-parent situation, with my mother. My father went to Canada because he didn't want to pay the alimony and child support."

I asked Eddie if it had been hard coming out to his family about his gayness. "I came out at nineteen. And even though my father wasn't really around, my mother called him, which I didn't understand. I said to her, 'What are you callin' *him* for?' " He laughed, recalling the scene. "I guess he was supposed to play Daddy."

Fortunately, Eddie isn't dependent on his family for financial support. "I had a little money saved, but not in a bank account. It's hidden in this apartment. And so when I got sick there was really no record that I had money and I didn't tell the agencies I had this money. Fortunately, my rent is nothing and besides, my roommate is sharing expenses. If he wasn't here, I don't know how I would be surviving. Because I only get $363 from Social Security, plus food stamps and Medicaid."

Because so many long-term survivors have mentioned the importance of religion, I asked Eddie how he felt. "I was raised Catholic," Eddie explained, "but now I'm not into organized religion. I see too much hypocrisy. I'm slightly religious, not overly religious. When it's my time to go, it's my time to go. I spent a month in Vermont on a farm. That's where I kind of got a spiritual awakening.

"Whoever God is, all he signifies to me is the whole spirit of everything—the whole universe. And to think that this is it—you're here, and you go, and then you never come back—doesn't make sense to me. Now, you may come back, but there may be other stops along the universe, you know? And maybe you will stop here again. I don't dwell on it too much. And in the meantime, I'm not here to judge people. I just do what I can. That's why I'm involved with the Minority Task Force.

"I was never politically active before. To me, working at the Task Force is more a spiritual thing. What you give, you get back. I can see it. Because there are all these people volunteering out there that don't have AIDS, and I see all the love and the beauty that they have and I want some of that. And I know that if I start giving that out, I'll get it back."

We discussed politics. I mentioned my theory that one of the reasons blacks and Hispanics die sooner than white gay men with AIDS had to do with the effects of poverty and racism. I asked him whether he felt that as a black man, he had gotten less than the best health care. "Actually, no," he said. "Not at all. The reason I think blacks and Hispanics don't do so well with AIDS is because in the minority community, AIDS is about IV drug use. IV drug users obviously aren't taking care of themselves. I'm talking about the ones that are on *drugs,* honey! They're addicted to drugs. And the survival statistics basically are dealing with not the gay blacks, or gay Hispanics. It's basically dealing with the IV community."

Eddie wanted to make sure I didn't think he was blaming anyone for having AIDS. In fact, he gets angry when anyone talks about blame. "My grandfather, who's kind of a bigot, said, 'Oh, take all drug addicts and kill them off or put them in jail.' And I said, 'How can you say that?' We got into an argument. I said, 'They're no different than you sitting here drinking alcohol. It's all drugs. I told him, 'The reason you drink is because there's something in you that needs to alter that specific moment; and some people are trying to erase or cover up more than just a specific moment.' "

"What is the solution?" I asked.

"I believe the drug thing can be worked out," he said. "And I believe in psychotherapy. Like you go to the dentist, you go to a psychotherapist."

Eddie was finding therapy helpful. "I just started, actually, but I'm optimistic that it will help." And echoing his basic approach to AIDS— and to life—he said, "I don't have anything to lose."

Eddie clearly believes the mind is a powerful healing tool. "I've done meditation and visualization. And I have some subliminal tapes. It calms your mind, your subconscious. Actually, your subconscious is what controls who you are anyway and the reactions that you have. I do visualizations. It's like a cartoon animation. It shows you how the body's immune system works. I can't say it hasn't helped, because I'm doing quite well."

I asked Eddie why he thought he was living beyond predictions. "Because I'm optimistic!" he said, without a moment's hesitation. "AIDS also helped me change my attitudes, change my frame of mind. The reason that I feel I'm doing well is not just because of the AZT, but because I'm optimistic."

I asked him how he manages to sustain his optimism in the face of a relentless campaign of negativity about AIDS. He said he doesn't bother reading negative propaganda about how AIDS is invariably fatal. "That's just somebody's opinion, and I'm not gonna let it affect me," he stated emphatically. "I was always a sick child. I had polio. I had real bad allergies, and it didn't affect me that negatively.

"When I was in the hospital recently, I looked really bad," Eddie admitted. "I had lost a lot of weight. Everybody was talking about, 'Hey, Eddie's dying.' I really don't think about whether or not I'll die from AIDS," he explained. "But I *don't* look at it as a death warrant; I see it as an awakening. In fact, I feel a little more fortunate than a lot of the motherfuckers out there, because it makes me take the time to look and see the flowers. Everybody walks around here in a fog, you know? It's not the quantity, it's the quality. That's my attitude."

Like other survivors, Eddie took his diagnosis as a sign to start living, not to start dying. "When I got out of the hospital, the first thing I did was, I went to Venezuela! And not for any AIDS cure; I went for a *head* cure—to soak up the sun. I just said, 'Fuck it; I'm going."

Why Venezuela?

"Because I'd never been to Venezuela," he said, laughing.

I asked Eddie what advice, besides visiting Venezuela, he'd give to someone like him who wanted to become a long-term survivor.

"First off, be optimistic. Because to me a lot of people suffer from stress. They think, 'I'm dying.' And 'This is the end.' And 'Why me?' I say, 'Act positive! Deal with it! Take the first step and deal with it. Then be good to yourself. Treat yourself. Realize you're not immortal. You might not be here tomorrow, so have a good time today.' And when I say have a good time, it's not like abuse yourself. It's not like, 'I may not be here tomorrow, so fuck it.'

"Basically, I would advise someone to go on AZT. What do you have to lose? If they're going to monitor you and they see that there's a reaction, then they'll take you off. Because there're other things that they can try now."

Eddie has absolutely no patience for negativity. He challenges it whenever he encounters it. "Just the other day, this Haitian guy called up the Minority Task Force and he was tripping out. He hadn't been to the doctor in a long time. And he'd start crying and then he'd hang up the phone and then he'd call back. He wouldn't give any information about where he lived or nothing. So I spoke to him and I said, 'Hey, I'm a PWA myself.' I have a certain frankness when I talk. I could say, 'Hey, you're not the only one in this boat. There's a lot of people on this boat, and the first step is learning to take care of yourself.' And he said, 'Oh, isn't there no hope?' I said, 'What do you mean, there's no hope? If there's no hope, you'd be dead already.'" Eddie laughed. He told me that he explained to the distraught man that he now had the opportunity to *do* something to make himself healthier. "I told him," Eddie said, "it's not the quantity, it's the quality. And I believe it truly is."

RON

"Basically, doing what I love is my therapy."

▨▨▨ Most PWAs realize that your chances of becoming a long-term survivor are better if you have KS than if you have had PCP or other opportunistic infections. But I knew at least one long-term survivor who had had PCP six years ago. He had been very involved in the early PWA activist movement. Unfortunately, he declined to be interviewed for the book. He was afraid that even if he told his story using a pseudonym, someone might recognize him and he would suffer further discrimination. He had long since left the activist movement and moved to New Jersey and was living a quiet life far from the maddening AIDS crowd. I was disappointed, but I understood and respected his reasons for declining.

Fortunately, while on my way to interview a long-term survivor with KS, I literally bumped into a long-term survivor of PCP, who was himself scurrying distractedly up Eighth Avenue. I had met Ron (who asked that I not use his last name) a year earlier in my capacity as editor of the PWA *Newsline*. As I apologized for bumping into him, I mentioned my book and the dilemma I was facing. "There don't seem to be any long-term survivors of PCP," I complained. He smiled devilishly and said, "Oh, yes there are. Me."

Ron and I are about the same age and we have a lot in common. For instance, we are both escapees from small-town small-mindedness. (It sometimes seems to me that every third homosexual living on either coast is a fugitive from the Midwest.) During our interview, I learned that we also had similar fast-lane histories: "The St. Marks Baths. The Everhard. Parties. Lofts. The Mineshaft. The Saint on Saturday nights. The whole scene. I was," he says, searching for the right euphemism, "very . . . social."

Ron, however, had outdone me in the controlled-substances category.

"I used a lot of drugs. The designer drugs. I think we all shopped at the same place, where you came out with a little shopping bag. . . ." He giggled.

But AIDS changed all that. He recounted the start of his AIDS odyssey. "In December 1983, I was very, very sick. I was bronchoscoped, and they diagnosed pneumocystis. Prior to that I had had problems with shingles, bronchitis, and rashes."

Ron firmly believes that stress is a major contributor to AIDS and that getting rid of stress in one's life is an important part of any survival strategy. "At the point I was diagnosed with PCP, I was working as an executive in a high-stress design job. And my lover and I were on the verge of breaking up. But my AIDS diagnosis seemed to bring us together."

Like many long-term survivors, he decided to quit his stressful job and do what he had always longed to do: paint and travel. "We were planning to retire to Paris. I thought I would paint until . . ." Until. His goal of becoming a long-term survivor hadn't gelled in his mind yet. "I wanted the happy *rainbow* story," he joked.

As for most long-term survivors, the crisis of AIDS forced an emotional housecleaning. Without consciously planning to, Ron made changes in most of his relationships. Coming out as a PWA to his family was extremely difficult. "I wanted to tell them I was moving to Paris. I hadn't really planned to tell them that I was sick, but I decided that if it came up, I wouldn't deny it. They knew that I had been in the hospital. The very first night home, they guessed. They just asked me: 'Do you have AIDS?' "

With delightfully droll theatrics, Ron acted out the scene for me. "This led to two weeks of trauma. I just sat on the bed reading the Bible, because somehow, that was what I felt I should be doing at their house. There was *lots* of yelling, screaming, and arguments." His eyes rolled gaily heavenward as he laughed riotously. "It was all very 'Where did we go wrong?' "

After a lot of hard work, relations with his family have become more manageable. "We've worked out a lot of our difficulties, but they will never accept my life-style. But at least they are really trying. We're on friendly terms."

The soap opera with his family was raising his stress level; more was in store. "My lover was supposed to be getting ready for the move, subletting the apartment, etc. But two weeks later, when I came back to New York, I discovered I was being *evicted*. I found out that during my stay in the hospital, although I was receiving full salary, none of my bills had been paid! All my money had gone up his nose with cocaine! I now had $15,000 in debts, and 74 cents in the bank. I had to kick him out and change the locks." (The lyrics to Gloria Gaynor's disco hit, "I Will Survive," floated through my brain: "I should have changed that stupid lock, I should have made you leave your key. . . .")

"It was horrible. We'd been together for two years, but I never knew that he had a coke problem. But he just went crazy at the time—crazy, I think, because of my diagnosis. It just sent him into the deep end."

Luckily, at this low point in Ron's life, his physician suggested that he see a therapist. "It was the best thing that ever happened to me. It changed my whole outlook. The therapist helped me get off the Valium they'd given me in the hospital." His physician also started him on two double-strength Bactrim daily, to prevent another occurrence of PCP. This, Ron believes, is a major reason why he's still alive today.

Ron has a wonderful relationship with his doctor. Far ahead of the current vogue, Ron's doctor prescribed acyclovir—an antiherpes medication. Ron had chosen not to take AZT. "My doctors say, 'Oh, you're doing so well. Why screw it up?' "

Slowly but surely, Ron began to take control of his life. Like many PWAs, he combined allopathic and alternative approaches: "Bactrim and macrobiotics," he quipped. "I started checking into nutrition and I put myself on a macrobiotic diet. And I started exercising as much as I could and drawing, because I'd read books like *Getting Well Again* by the Simontons. I also read Louise Hay and started getting interested in that sort of thing.

As with many other long-term survivors, the New Age held great attraction for Ron. "I was really very strict, very—total macro, total health nut—for a year. I really saw what a difference it made. But I'm no longer macrobiotic. I couldn't live that way. I'm not going to torture myself. I mean, there are other ways of torturing myself. But to be antisocial and to only eat brown rice and roots . . ." He grinned. "I'm not going to do it. In fact, I've slipped back to having a drink occasionally. And I do smoke cigarettes. Basically, I just have a good time. I eat better than I ever did, I still get a lot of rest, I exercise, and I'm going to the shrink."

Ron didn't set out to be a long-term survivor. In fact, "The first six months were horrible. A nightmare. I didn't know who I was, what was going to happen." But about a year after his diagnosis with PCP and AIDS, it suddenly dawned on him: "Okay. No one else is going to heal me; it's up to me!"

AIDS was a turning point for Ron. Like others, he simply reinvented his life. "Everyone else was gone from my life. I decided that I didn't want to deal with them. And I really focused on *me*, what *I* wanted to do—like painting. I developed a technique of drawing for myself by doing deep-breathing exercises, which I'd picked up in yoga class, and doing that while I drew."

Ron then decided to reach out to other PWAs. "I started teaching the art therapy program at Metropolitan-Duane Center for Mental Health and I was in on the early meetings of the PWA Coalition in New York."

Eventually, Ron decided to pull back from his political involvement. "I decided to focus on returning to a normal way of life. I had spent three years being an 'AIDS person,' and I decided that I could either go on being an 'AIDS person' or try to be a person who happens to have AIDS. So I moved aside and started focusing on my artwork—and me."

This strategy continues to work for Ron, who, like so many other long-term survivors, claims to be happier now than ever before. "My life is so much better and fulfilling. Yes, I worry and I get very scared. I think about death a lot. At first, I was afraid. I thought about dying from AIDS, but I never really believed it. I knew it was a possibility. But I don't believe I'm going to die of AIDS."

Ron said that media assertions that AIDS is 100 percent fatal don't really bother him. "I just don't think that's correct. Sure, we probably will all die—thirty years from now. And I'm sure they'll say, 'At *last!* He *finally* died of AIDS.' "

My overwhelming impression of Ron was one of optimism tempered by realism. "I read the paper every morning to find out if some break-through has happened. I get excited about new drugs," he said. "But on the other hand, I'm not a person who's going to rush out and take an experimental drug."

Ron continues to comfortably blend an allopathic and a holistic approach to surviving AIDS: "I'm on Bactrim, I'm on a full regimen of vitamins, I exercise, and I meditate. Basically, doing what I love doing is my therapy."

And speaking of love, Ron reminded me that I had introduced him to another PWA at one of the singles' tea socials that I run. The relationship was a bust, but Ron explained that after a long period of abstinence, he was once again having sex—"safe sex, of course. I would *love* to have a lover. But this time around, it's got to be a *good* one," he laughed.

I asked Ron whether he thought about the possibility of life after death. He spoke movingly about his spirituality: "When I was a child, I was very religious, more so than my parents. But after discovering that I was gay, I stopped going to church. When I was diagnosed, I suddenly found myself going to Catholic and Episcopal churches, which is very strange for me. But I was going to try everything. I'd pray in Catholic churches.

I was constantly crying and going to the church. It wasn't so much for the church as it was just the thought of putting myself in this place of beauty and sitting there and thinking. That did me a lot of good.

"I do not go to church anymore. I went to a meeting once on AIDS and this Episcopal priest was preaching that people with AIDS are trash—slime from the depths of degradation and prostitutes—that sort of connotation. Which really aggravated me. I swore I would never go back there.

"I have found more spirituality through reading about Eastern philosophy and yoga and meditation and looking at my background. I'm a Cherokee Indian. I consider myself to be more of a New Age person who happens to believe in Christ—in a higher power. I believe there's life after death. It may be up in heaven or it may be that we come back and be a sofa or something. . . ." He laughed. "I don't know."

Asked to sum up his own sense of why he has beat the odds, Ron sighed deeply. "Oh, loving myself. Taking care of myself. Getting rid of a lot of guilt—guilt about sex, about who I am. Just loosening up and being me. And loving who I am. Being happy. Oh, and Bactrim, for preventing me from getting another bout of PCP."

I asked Ron what advice he would give to someone diagnosed fifteen minutes ago. After thoughtful consideration, he said, "Well, first things first: I would tell them to buy Louise Hay's books and tapes. I would advise checking out macrobiotics, taking a yoga class, and getting a shrink. And Bactrim to prevent PCP. Those are the immediate things to do. And don't take any experimental drugs. Just say 'no' to drugs unless your doctor says you have to. Then find out what you want to do with the rest of your life and go do it. Don't sit around and wait. Don't let anything stop you. Don't let money stop you, because it'll come. Believe. Believe in yourself. Believe that you can heal. That you have choices. That you can make the choices. That you have the power to determine what will happen."

"I love life. *I love life!*" he repeated with fervor, like some forties screen goddess. "I'm very proud of myself. I think I can do anything now."

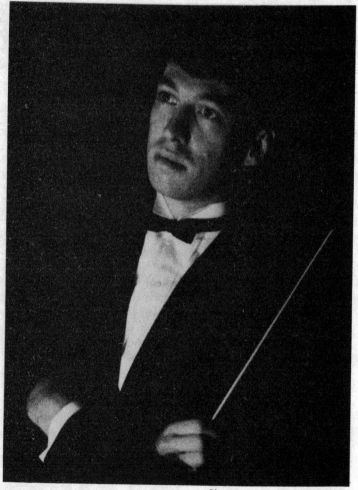

David Schofield.

DAVID SCHOFIELD

"Not everyone dies from AIDS."

▨▨▨ Within a week of interviewing Ron, I again struck gold in my search for long-term survivors of PCP. During a checkup, the pulmonary specialist who had bronchoscoped me for suspected PCP in 1982 agreed to give my phone number to her star patient, who eventually called me. David is more than a patient to this doctor; he and she had developed an extraordinarily close relationship. An accomplished organist, David even played at her wedding.

I met David in the imposing Gothic cathedral very near the hospital where we'd both spent so much sick time. Although technically I was meeting him at his job (he's the church's music director), I felt as if I were meeting him at his home, because his relationship to the church was so special. When he had been released from the hospital, frail and poor, the church had housed him and provided him with food and spiritual sustenance during his difficult recovery.

David was initially standoffish, for a very respectable reason: I had told him I wanted to use our interview for an article for the *Village Voice.* David felt the *Voice* had degenerated into a rag full of sad, self-consciously clever, ax-grinding reportage. My association with it was off-putting to him. But when I delightedly seconded his opinion of the *Voice,* the ice began to melt.

Originally, David had insisted on anonymity. But for reasons that will be explained later, he subsequently asked me to use his real, full name.

It turned out that David and I have a lot in common. We are roughly the same age, are both skeptical about experts, and are both musicians. David was AIDS Class of '83 and I was Class of '82. As of Halloween 1987, when our interview took place, David had survived AIDS and PCP for an amazing four years.

"In 1983 I was diagnosed with gonorrhea, hepatitis, mononucleosis, cytomegalovirus, and then pneumocystis pneumonia," he recited with clinical dispassion. "And after that, bronchial pneumonia and various other sundry . . ."—he paused to grope for the right word, then, laughing, said—"*minor* complications. I've never gotten PCP again, although I've had bronchial pneumonia three times since."

His admission that he has never taken any form of PCP prophylaxis, even though he is among those lucky enough to tolerate the powerful prophylactic antibiotics that so many PWAs are allergic to, surprised me. I asked why he didn't believe in prophylaxis.

"I only heard about prophylaxis in 1986. And at that time I was in very good health and I didn't want to mess things up. I thought I'd just leave things alone." David has also avoided enrolling in experimental protocols and eschews the unapproved drugs popular in the AIDS "underground." "I was examined by Dr. Lange last Wednesday, and he was very interested in the fact that I'd been taking tetracycline or erythromycin continuously for the last ten years for an ongoing acne condition. He felt that that probably had something to do with my ability to recover."

Although it seemed contradictory coming from someone who had taken antibiotics virtually nonstop for ten years for an acne condition, David expressed a holistic distrust of drugs: "I'm kind of horrified that when you go into the hospital they give you this for this and that for that, and they never question what the total effect is on your body of having all these different chemicals suddenly coming into it. I have a feeling that sometimes it's more detrimental than helpful."

Like me, David had vowed to avoid ever being bronchoscoped again. Being "bronched," as it's called in PWA slang, is an extremely unpleasant procedure where a tube containing a tiny TV camera is pushed down your throat and into your lung. Although one is Demeroled to within an inch of ecstasy, my memory is primarily one of drowning; one's throat is continually flushed with liquid anesthetic. In addition, one is vaguely aware of a horrific zinging sound, reminiscent of piano wire being scratched with a penny. Each time you hear the sound, little pinchers rip a tiny piece of your lung for a biopsy sample. Between the metallic zipping sound and the indescribable internal pinch, the experience is vaguely like being bitten by a mosquito on the *inside* of your lungs. We both shuddered at the memory.

Now, each time David gets symptoms of pneumonia, he insists on being treated presumptively with powerful antibiotics; and each time, the symptoms have resolved. I hypothesized that in a way, his frequent on-again/off-again use of antibiotics functions as a sort of PCP prophylaxis.

David cooperates good-naturedly whenever AIDS researchers want to try to find the secret of his success. "I guess I'm sort of a guinea pig," he laughed. "But that's all right, because it would be great if they could find something that could help others."

I asked him if he dabbled with holistic approaches to healing. "Acupuncture and acupressure have my respect. If my doctor thought it might be beneficial for me, I might try it. But I'm very skeptical of the other things, such as the health food approach and multivitamins. That sort of thing doesn't interest me."

Though David rejects such New Age approaches as Louise Hay, he said that spirituality was an important part of his healing strategy. "About a year and a half before I was diagnosed with AIDS, my sense of religion and spiritual life was awakening, and I was becoming interested in the church and in church work. I was raised a Baptist; in fact, my father was a Baptist minister. But I converted to Roman Catholic. So I had been pretty well firmly planted in it by the time I got AIDS.

"I think that the spirit is one of the most important factors—in my case in particular. The people in my church were extremely supportive. Before and after my hospitalization from pneumocystis I was given a room in the rectory and was brought food from the cook every day. I lived here for about two months, because I couldn't do anything for myself. The maids would come and clean my room and people from the church came and visited me."

In addition to the extraordinary outpouring of care and concern from his church, David received love and support from his lover, his friends, and family. "My parents were very supportive. They even came to see me, and I just knew that everybody was with me, and that was a tremendous lift. So that accounts for a lot, I think."

I discovered that two more things David and I had in common were our Hoosier heritage and our past sex lives. David considered himself to have been a fairly typical urban gay man of the late seventies. "But I never was big on drugs. I had had a drinking problem early on, but that was over by the time I moved to New York from Indiana. But sex was a big deal in my life." Raising his eyebrows for emphasis, he said, laughing: "I had a *lot* of sex.

"When the Centers for Disease Control asked me to estimate my lifetime number of sex partners for some study they were doing, I hesitated. And they said, 'Well . . . fifty?' And I said, 'Oh, *no. Many* more than that.' And they said, 'Well, one hundred?' And I said, 'No, probably more like in the thousands somewhere, you know?' " He laughed again, unselfconsciously. "It raised their eyebrows, but they wrote it down."

Although it often confuses those with limited imagination, David managed to rack up thousands of sexual partners while maintaining a primary, committed relationship. "I was in my present relationship when I was diagnosed. We've been lovers since 1979. Our agreement was that we could go out and do what we pleased as long as neither of us took these people's names and phone numbers. In other words, no affairs!

"Of course, since my illness, that has changed some. My sex life certainly has changed very much. Not to say I haven't had sex; I just don't have unsafe sex anymore.

"I remember that the nurse at the hospital told me, 'You know, you can still . . .' She was talking specifically about me and my lover, that, you know, we could still have sex the way we always had. She didn't think it would be a problem. I thought she was crazy!"

I asked him the $64,000 question: Why did he think he was alive so long after his PCP diagnosis?

"That's a great mystery. I suppose that there are still things left for me to do on this earth that I haven't done. I believe that there is a God and that his purpose for me on this earth is not completed."

At the time of our interview, David was selective about who he told about his diagnosis. "If it's someone who is fairly close to me, it's my nature to bare all and just be truthful. Still, I don't think everybody needs to know. But I've never had any problem with discrimination."

I asked him if his decision to recuperate from PCP at the church had economic motivations. "I've had real money problems. I have no insurance. I was on Medicaid and social security. When I began to work again, my Medicaid was cut off, of course. And the money that I was making from my job was not nearly enough to pay for the medical attention that I needed. Again, people at my church and my friends were very supportive, monetarily this time. My doctor sees me for free. This is partly, I think, because at this point my case is interesting, and, she's just a wonderful woman.

"During my second hospitalization—the time that I was diagnosed with PCP—the social services at the hospital had not given me all the forms to fill out to apply for Medicaid, so my Medicaid hadn't gone through. My second admission was about a month after the first one, so I had this ten-thousand-dollar bill that was unpaid. And I was wheeled into the admitting office in a wheelchair with 104-degree fever, gasping for breath. And this administrator from behind the desk said that I couldn't be admitted because I owed them ten thousand dollars and that I would have to pay the ten thousand dollars before they could possibly admit me. They kept me there for three hours. Finally, the friend who was with me raised holy hell and they admitted me through the emergency room. But that was really not very nice."

Although he signed up for the services of the Gay Men's Health Crisis, David avoided support groups. "I really didn't feel the need to join a support group. I did go to the recreation group once, but I was not very happy with that occasion, so I never went again. But I have used them for referrals for doctors and that sort of thing."

Then he told me an amazing story that seemed to contradict his assertion that he didn't need to be around other PWAs. "I do volunteer work at the hospital and regularly visit AIDS patients. The person who runs the visitation program told me I'm not supposed to tell them that I have AIDS."

I gasped. "Why?"

"Actually, I think it's for the best, because what we do is really just visit them in the hospital and shoot the breeze; we're not supposed to become buddies. But there's no way you can do that and not become close to people. There are some people that I just hit it off with. I became very close to one guy in particular. I came to his room every day, sometimes twice, and sometimes three times a day toward the end. I slept in his room. I changed his bed and washed him for five months. And finally he died."

"And in all that time," I asked incredulously, "you never told him you had AIDS?"

"Actually, I did eventually tell him, and it really surprised him. But it was a good thing in a way. At the time that I told him, he was sort of despondent. I gave him . . ."

He paused, in painful recollection, and, as is my bad habit, I finished his sentence: "Hope?"

"Yes, hope," he said quietly. "Exactly. It gave him hope to think that there are people who can rise above this."

I asked him if he had assumed he was going to die of AIDS or whether he had set out to be a long-term survivor.

"I never have asked my doctors how long I had to live. But they kept listing all these diseases that people with AIDS were susceptible to. And so I finally asked, 'Well, what if, you know, I get pneumocystis again, or KS?' And the answer was usually, 'You die.'

"It was just a little bit scary at first and then basically I said, 'Well, if it happens it happens.' And I had almost died from PCP. Actually, the doctors were rather surprised that I didn't die. And surviving PCP was a great experience and has changed a lot of my thinking and views on life. Many things that seemed *terribly* important don't really seem very important now. It's changed the way that I look at people in general and changed the way that I deal with people, that I think about myself, that I think about death, and that I think about living and I think about life after death. There *is* life after death. I'm absolutely positive of it, after having that near-death experience. I didn't have a vision; I just had a sense. . . . I was sort of in a transitory state for a while and I couldn't . . . I mean, I wasn't in the next world, but I could sense it."

Unlike survivor Steven Pieters, David's near-death experience had a disquieting effect. "Actually, I long to be there," he sighed.

⊠ At the time of our interview, David said that he didn't feel any responsibility to be a role model. But after I published a transcript of my interview with him in a PWA publication, he sent me the following beautiful note explaining why he had now decided to "come out" as a long-term AIDS survivor:

> *Dear Michael:*
>   *I was very pleased to see you could use my interview. Your article was great. As a fellow long-term survivor I could really relate to your problems. Although until very recently I've been reluctant to be public about my AIDS diagnosis (PCP, 1983). I too have had the problem of people not believing my diagnosis which is a little flattering ("You look so good") but also irritating. If I'm not dead or on death's doorstep, then maybe I really didn't have AIDS. . . . When I tell them I've got AIDS, people say things like "You mean you're HIV positive, don't you?" or "You mean ARC, right?" AIDS or ARC, who cares? What do these people want? That I should get sick to prove I'm really a PWA?*
>   *It's a head trip and a dangerous one because sometimes I find myself buying into their sick expectations.*
>   *But now I have decided to keep my guard up against these attitudes. They're as lethal as any virus!*
>   *It's taken me a long time to be able to do this or know it's necessary, but I'm coming out of the AIDS closet and I'm signing my full name to this and if there is another issue of the* Newsline, *I hope you'll publish it. I regret having done our interview under a pseudonym.*
>   *I have been a person with AIDS for five years now and am still going strong. I don't say this to brag (I'm certainly not superhuman), but so that anyone who might read this will know that NOT EVERYONE DIES FROM AIDS!*
>   *I hope I don't have to go to the length you did to prove it.*
>   *Yours,*
>   *David Schofield*

GARY MACKLER

⊠⊠⊠ Although the CDC's study on long-term survivors indicates that there are individuals who developed AIDS as the result of IV drug use who have survived for three or more years, I was not able to find any. But because I felt strongly that the struggle of IVDUs with AIDS to survive AIDS needed to be told, I decided to include interviews with individuals who had survived significantly beyond the predictions for IVDUs with AIDS. At the time of our interview in November 1987, Gary had survived for eighteen months.

I met the amazing Gary Mackler and his lifemate, Joy Chiavetta, through the PWA Health Group. Gary, a very handsome, quiet, heterosexual, former IV drug-using PWA, eventually joined the board of directors of the PWA Coalition. His butch expertise as a construction worker became invaluable when the coalition decided to renovate and move into a building in Chelsea.

Joy and Gary first met in grade school. They fell in love in 1980, the year Gary entered a drug treatment program. I interviewed them in their Chelsea high-rise apartment in late November 1987 and discovered that there were aspects to Gary's personality that I'd never encountered during our tenure as fellow Coalition board members. As I was to discover, only those lucky enough to get close to him ever saw more than one side, and I think that only Joy got to see all the fascinating aspects of Gary Mackler.

Gary was the first self-acknowledged IV drug user I had ever gotten to know. Like many other Americans, I had a stereotypical view of what an IV drug user "should" be like, and Gary shattered every myth. He was disarmingly frank about his drug history and appropriately proud of having beaten drugs.

Like many IV drug users, Gary was not unacquainted with illness. "I had had chronic, active hepatitis B; non-A, non-B hepatitis; and mononucleosis a couple of times. When I went into the drug treatment program, I immediately went into the hospital, because I was jaundiced. A couple of years after that, I started hearing terms like 'compromised immune system.' I was really tired, but I was working and going to school. I wondered if my symptoms were only my imagination."

During our interview, Gary was running a low-grade temperature and was feeling generally miserable. Looking back from the vantage point of a diagnosis of full-blown AIDS, he recalled frequently feeling as lousy as he did that day and wondered whether he hadn't really had AIDS long before his official diagnosis. He smiled at a recollection of those more carefree, pre-AIDS days: "I had one doctor five years ago who looked at my blood work and told me, 'What you need to do is get married and settle down and you'll be fine.' "

He first heard the diagnosis of AIDS-Related Complex applied to him in 1984, but he wasn't really worried. "Looking back, I have had symptoms of what would now be called ARC at least since 1980. For years I was told that 'this will probably not get worse.' Doctors just kept saying, 'Well, you have these symptoms because of your history of hepatitis.' It was easier to keep calling it 'chronic active hepatitis' than AIDS. And there didn't appear to be anything I could do about my immune deficiency, in any case.

"But actually, I already knew," he said. "I mean, it was anticlimactic when I got my HIV antibody test results, because it was so clear what was going on. I was sick for a long, long time, with fevers as high as 104, 105. I had diarrhea and was losing weight every day. Of course, I always held out the hope that it wasn't AIDS, but I wasn't surprised to find out in April of '85 that I was HIV positive. After that, my doctor gave me my ARC diagnosis."

In November 1984, Gary had been hospitalized with an intestinal infection that turned out to be campylobacter colitis. "The doctor said that he had never seen a case like mine," Gary recalled. During this hospitalization, Gary met Dr. Michael Lange, one of the world's foremost AIDS experts: "I guess Dr. Lange was really the first one to seriously suggest that my problems might be HIV-related."

Although the intestinal infection responded to antibiotics, Gary got steadily sicker and sicker. "At the end of April '86, I had candida in my mouth. And I started being short of breath. Looking back, we now know that I had an unusual case of PCP developing—unusual in that it began in the left lung only. Ninety-five percent of the time, from what I've been told, PCP develops in both lungs. So, when an X ray only showed a little something on the left lung, they said, 'Well, it's probably not PCP.' So the farce continued for another two months."

Joy seemed angrier than Gary at the runaround they'd gotten from the doctors over whether his problems were AIDS-related or not. But Gary reminded Joy that it wouldn't be fair to only blame the doctors. "There was also a certain denial on my part," Gary admitted. "I would wake up one day with a dry hacking cough; but then the next day, I wouldn't cough at all. So on the days when I felt okay, I was able to say, 'Well, there's really nothin' goin' on.' But it is true that I wasn't getting a lot of encouragement from the doctor to think anything different."

Finally, Gary's shortness of breath demanded that he be hospitalized. On June 1, 1986, a bronchoscopy confirmed the worst: pneumocystis carinii pneumonia and, therefore, AIDS. Because his PCP had been allowed to progress untreated for several months, Gary faced a tough battle to survive his first AIDS-defining infection. This was only the first of many life-threatening episodes that Gary would survive with the help of sheer grit.

Another problem was that Gary tended to suffer tremendous side effects from many of his medications. "During my first bout with PCP, I don't know how I tolerated the Bactrim, but somehow I did. I was kind of delirious for about a week. I had blinding headaches and the light really bothered my eyes. They thought for a while that I must have CMV of the brain."

Eventually, Gary recovered and was released from the hospital. But the best thing to come out of that hospitalization was that Gary met Dr. Don Kotler, an AIDS expert who was to become a good friend as well as Gary's primary physician. Gary spoke in reverential tones about the extraordinary relationship he developed with his doctor.

"Don Kotler was very pragmatic. He said: 'You have AIDS.' He didn't minimize the seriousness of it, but he didn't maximize it. He never said, 'You have this amount of time to live.' His attitude was, 'Well, let's see what we can do about today.' "

Kotler's bedside manner was in sharp contrast to the approach of several other doctors, who had told Gary and Joy that the average survival time for an IV drug user with AIDS was only nine months. I asked how the pronouncement of such a death sentence had affected them.

"I want to pick my words very carefully here," Gary said in the quiet, thoughtful way he always spoke. "Joy, you can help me with this a little bit. I developed an attitude that was pretty fatalistic, you know? I got into . . . well, it was almost like a mystical frame of mind. I don't know if I'm describing it accurately, but I was almost nostalgic and romantic about death. I wanted to do some traveling and I wanted to go back to some places where I'd had some good times. It wasn't a defeatist attitude, but it wasn't like 'Well, let me get on with my life now and do what I can' either. Thinking about it now, it was so much bullshit. But that didn't last long. I quickly got back into that 'Let me live my life and continue to do the best I can' frame of mind."

Gary smiled lovingly at Joy and said, "Joy had *no* patience for me during this period—no patience for this otherworldly stuff. She was like, 'Oh, get *real* already.'

"I may eventually die from AIDS; I don't deny that. But actually it was more jarring to figure out that I also might *not* die from AIDS. After my hospitalization, my health stabilized for a while. And it was like, 'Well, what am I going to *do* with my life?' That was a very scary kind of limbo—a kind of never-never land of uncertainty."

It was during this period of uncertainty about how to *live* with AIDS that Gary happened to hear about the AIDS Mastery—a weekend workshop that helps people deal with AIDS and that turned out to be run by a person *with* AIDS—the one and only Max Navarre. (Max was a fellow board member of the PWA Coalition.)

"I was really skeptical," Gary recalled. "I went to an introductory meeting two days before the weekend, because I was aware of a certain sentiment in the holistic community which says that a person has, you know, 'caused' the disease to happen, or has control over the course of it. And I *really* would *not* hear that. So I figured I would ask them and they'd say, 'Well, yes, we believe that' and then I could walk out and not do it. But that's not what happened." His eyes twinkled.

"I was itching for a fight," he recalled. "But they answered my questions okay. And Joy and I did the Mastery and found it a really positive, life-affirming experience."

Aside from the insights he gained from the Mastery itself, Gary got something else from the experience: "I met handfuls of people who had been diagnosed three years ago and more." He also met his first self-empowered PWA, Max Navarre, and they began a wonderful friendship.

"There was an instant simpatico between Joy and me and Max. Max had had similar experiences with substance abuse, so I didn't feel so completely alone as an IV drug user among so many gay men. That can be very alienating. But here was someone who had been there, been through what I'd been through.

"Before the Mastery, I'd been pretty sure I was going to die soon, and I guess I was preparing for that. The Mastery really changed all that. I first heard about the possibility of living with AIDS from Max. After meeting him, my attitude changed. Not overnight, but I became more like I always had been before AIDS. I've *always* been a fighter—a very aggressive person."

"Gary had been a fighter since 1980, when he'd entered the drug treatment program," Joy proudly explained. "Even before he got sick he was already a voracious reader and was very well informed about a lot of things."

"I'd been pursuing what I believed my life should be *before* I got sick," Gary said. "Kicking drugs had given me a second chance at life. I actually had a kind of life plan. I had quit a job because I didn't want to spend my time doing something I didn't get anything out of. Life had already become too precious to me. I wanted to go back to school and study photography and writing. So when I was diagnosed, I didn't make any great discovery that 'Well, this is what life's all about.' "

Gary's fighting spirit expressed itself in extensive research into his treatment options. "Around '86, when I had the bacterial colitis," he said, "I was researching what treatments were available. I read, things like *AIDS Treatment News*, the treatment directory [put out by the American Foundation for AIDS Research]."

"Gary's mother is a librarian," Joy added. "And she started researching things for him."

Clearly, Gary was surrounded by many people who loved him ferociously and who pitched in to help him in his battle with AIDS.

After a lot of investigation, Gary decided to get on the AIDS treatment merry-go-round by entering an AZT protocol. Despite the fact that he fit the entry criteria, he was rejected twice. But he persisted and eventually began taking AZT.

"I wasn't thrilled with taking it. And I expressed my concerns about it to Dr. Kotler. Although he felt that it was something that I should do, I made the decision for myself. I wasn't sure that AZT was a good thing, but I felt that I should either decide *not* to take it and be happy with that decision, or to take it and not be half-assed about that decision. And eventually, I decided to take it."

Even after he started taking AZT, he kept his ears to the ground for word of other, less toxic treatments. This led to an amazing adventure that Gary believes saved his life. "In the waiting room of Roosevelt Hospital, I first heard about AL721—egg lipids—and about the Weizmann Institute in Israel, which had developed AL721, and about a letter in *the New England Journal of Medicine* about AL721 blocking HIV. I also heard through the PWA grapevine that an eight-person lipid study was being done right there at St. Luke's/Roosevelt Hospital." Again, however, he was told that he didn't qualify for that study, even though he had AIDS. "But the doctor told me off the record, 'You're a walking time bomb. If I were you, I'd get on a plane to Israel.'"

Gary was excited about the possibility of getting this new treatment, but his confidant, Dr. Kotler, discouraged him from flying to Israel.

At the time Gary decided to try lipids he had been recovering slowly from his latest AIDS complication—cryptosporidium, the same debilitating disease that I had had. At his worst point, his weight had dropped from 145 down to a dangerous 115 pounds. Dr. Kotler had started him on hyperimmunized cow's milk, an experimental treatment for cryptosporidium. "Actually," Gary said proudly, "it was because I'd already been lucky once with an experimental treatment—the cow's milk had cured me of crypto—that I figured, why not lipids?" Dr. Kotler told Gary he thought it would be next to impossible to get lipids. That was just the kind of challenge that Gary loved to rise to. Gary recounted the fateful scene where he decided to go for broke in pursuit of egg lipids: "I remember we were all in my parents' kitchen—me, Joy, my parents, and my brother. My brother speaks Hebrew, so he called the doctor in Israel—even though, as it turned out, I didn't need a translator. I gave the doctor my medical history. Then I opened my heart to him, and I said, 'Look, what I'm asking you for is a chance to live. This is really what I want. I have a great zest and appreciation for life and I'm asking you to help me to be able to live it.'"

Joy and I watched him in silent admiration as he relived this powerful moment in his life. "It was like this bizarre, almost Fellini-esque kind of thing," he said, laughing. "My parents and my brother were at the window with their backs to me, and Joy was sitting on the floor. *And everyone was crying.* But no one wanted to make noise, because it was a long-distance connection."

Gary's heartfelt plea succeeded. The doctor agreed to treat Gary with egg lipids if he came to Israel. "I was on a plane that next Saturday—along with my whole family. My father was able to lay out the $10,000 that it cost for everyone to go to Israel, but I have paid him back," he said proudly. "I was really sick *before* I got on the airplane, and the fourteen-hour plane ride was real torture—both coming and going."

Gary had had to consider the logistics of traveling with a catheter implanted in his chest. Although his weight loss had stopped thanks to the cow's milk, he was still receiving TPN (total parenteral nutrition) and round-the-clock IV-drip.

"I had to travel to Israel with all my IV equipment," Gary recalled. "At the time I did it, though, I didn't think about it. It was like, 'Well, this is what you have to do,' and so I did it. Looking back, it's kind of staggering what we did—we meaning me, Joy, and my family. I'm not patting myself on the back, but *I* did it. I got myself there. It just didn't seem to me that *not* going was an option. There was no reason not to try. I was going to Israel and I was going to get AL721."

Gary must really have impressed the Israeli doctor, because he did something unheard of: The doctor made a house call—or a hotel call, as it were. "The first thing he told me was, 'You have the gift of hope.' " The doctor then insisted that Gary stop all other medications, including the AZT and the dapsone he was taking to prevent a recurrence of PCP. "He thought that AL721 was all that anyone needed," Gary recalled. Gary was absolutely unwilling to risk another bout of PCP. So he did what many PWAs are forced to do by difficult doctors: He lied. "I kept taking my dapsone and just didn't tell him. But I did stop the AZT, which I'd only been taking for a week and a half."

While in Israel, Gary ate thirty to sixty grams of egg lipids daily. He was in frequent phone contact with Dr. Kotler back in the States. Dr. Kotler was extremely displeased that Gary had stopped taking AZT, so when Gary returned to America he resumed taking it. (He soon had to go to half-dose because of anemia.)

After nineteen days, he felt well enough to leave Israel. "I improved. The fevers were subsiding and when I did have them, they were much lower. My appetite was coming back and I was putting on some weight."

Gary returned to the States with a forty-day supply of lipids. "I was very anxious about running out," Gary explained, "but the doctor promised me that as long as I needed it, he would supply it. I guess he was getting AL721 from the Weizmann Institute, which invented it."

Gary's experience with lipids led to his involvement with the PWA Health Group. (Dr. Joe Sonnabend and fellow PWA Tom Hannan and I had founded the PWA Health Group to import and distribute egg lipids at cost for those PWAs who wanted them.) "I feel very fortunate that my family was able to support me, financially and emotionally, during that trip. On the other hand, I feel that it is the most horrible crime that I *had* to go to Israel. I blame the government and the regulatory agencies who are responsible—'irresponsible' is probably a better term—for seeing that promising treatments never reach those whom they may help. It has been almost two years to the day since Robert Gallo published his letter in *The New England Journal of Medicine* saying that lipids had shown promising results. It makes me very, very angry. That is why I was attracted to the PWA Health Group. The idea of a community-based group—a group of us PWAs—making policy on what will essentially be their fate makes a whole lot of sense to me."

Gary changed subjects and began to speak about his drug-using past. I wanted to talk about Gary's IV drug history, but I warned him that I knew little about that culture. I told him that if I asked anything stupid or offensive, he should feel free to tell me. Gary told me not to worry about it; he said he was quite comfortable talking about the dark days of his life and proceeded to tell his story.

"I started smokin' pot in '68 when I was twelve. Shortly thereafter, I got involved in, basically, pills and psychedelics—amphetamines, barbiturates, acid. I had dropped out of school in the tenth grade. And when I was fifteen, I left home and left New York City."

I asked him whether his drug use was part of the youth rebellion of the sixties or whether there were other reasons. Having just heard the moving tale of how his family rallied around him to help him save his life, I was startled to learn that his relationship with his family had not always been good.

"I had serious problems with my family," Gary explained. "When I was fourteen, there was serious talk about filing a PINS petition, which means 'Person in Need of Supervision.' My parents were going to go to the judge and say, 'We can't take care of him, so we want the state to take care of him.' And if the court says okay, you go to a juvenile facility. It was at this point that I left home.

"Drugs were more the result of *other* problems I was having at home. I had been arrested several times as a juvenile for possession, possession with intent, criminal sale. And there was some assault of some kind. I had been like floating around the country from the time I was fifteen until the time I was about twenty, when I got busted. I lived in California, Montana, Oregon, and Vermont, but mostly in Texas. I'd come back to New York, make some money, go back. But I basically came back for a good while when I was twenty."

As I sat trying to reconcile the sweet, gentle Gary I knew with the violent, drugged-out person he was describing, I saw waves of emotion wash over Joy as the man she loved recounted this painful period of his life.

"I got married," he said, matter-of-factly, "and it was at that time that I started getting *seriously* involved with drugs. I was strung out on all kinds of barbiturates, Quaaludes—you name it. I wasn't shooting drugs yet, but I was dealing. And I was also doing burglaries. Oh God," he said, "my life just started falling apart. Then I started shooting up with Percodan and Demerol, and eventually morphine and then heroin. And then

I started also shooting cocaine, which was the beginning of the end. My life was just coming apart at the seams. I almost died a couple of times through drug overdoses." He shook his head at the memory.

Gary commented on one of many of the paradoxes of his life. Part of his problem was that he was so good at what he did—even good at the bad things. "I had a very successful drug business. I had a *lot* of money. But . . . it's all gone now. I was finally arrested in a very large bust, and the cops took most of the $100,000 in cash I had. Also a lot of drugs and guns disappeared—never made it into evidence. But they left enough to have me arrested for a full-scale felony. It's not a pretty story," he recalled sadly.

I asked him whether he was aware of AIDS-related symptoms during this period. "During this whole time," he explained, "I went through de-tox three times. During one of them, they told me I had hepatitis."

At the time of our interview, Gary had already survived full-blown AIDS eighteen months—exactly twice the length he had been told that former IV drug users with AIDS survive. I asked Gary how he explained the fact that he was beating the odds for an IVDU with AIDS. He thought for a moment, then said, "Well, first of all, I'm seven years without using drugs. Besides that, I think that there's a *multitude* of reasons which have contributed to beating the odds. One is I have received aggressive, excellent health care—although I've had to fight for it. Another reason is that I have an incredible desire to live, and an incredible zest for life. It's just part of how I'm made up, to be active and doing something, and I'm currently taking a class in amateur photography. And I like to write.

"Another reason is that I've always been real scrappy—a hard-assed fighter. And I am also very angry. Maybe angry enough to stay alive," he laughed. "And I get a tremendous amount of unconditional love and support from Joy and my friends and family. How does someone do it who doesn't have all the love and support I have?

"There's a lot I have to live for," he said. "I think it's very important to be involved with things that give you pleasure. I have many passions— photography, music, writing. These things also sustain me."

I asked Gary whether he had been raised to be religious. "My brother's orthodox Jewish, and my mother's Jewish, and my father's an atheist. I'm kind of opposed to everything," he chuckled. "I don't believe in, you know, a higher form. I think that there's an order to the universe, and that that order is random chaos."

I laughed, but Gary was quite serious.

"That's really what I believe. There's something that I also feel very strongly about, and maybe this will illustrate it. I remember a TV show where a black woman IV drug user was being interviewed in the hospital. She was very sick and she was sobbing. And she said, 'You know, sometimes I wake up and I say "Lord, why me?" and then I think about all those things I did out in the street and I *know* why.' And I hate that. I hate that some people are encouraged to feel that they deserve AIDS, or that they deserve to have this virus. And I believe that that is so untrue. But whenever you talk about religions, that attitude of blame and guilt always rears its head—that we're paying a price for something. And that is so horrible and offensive to me."

Gary warmed to the subject of his absolute loathing of religion. I told him that it was a relief to meet a fellow long-term survivor who shared my contempt for religion.

"The concept of sin is very offensive to me," Gary explained.

"Gary doesn't understand faith at all," Joy said. "He questions everything and he defines religion as the absence of free thought."

Joy's religious views were not so harsh. She occasionally took comfort from talking to nuns and others who would visit Gary in the hospital. "Gary didn't begrudge me that kind of comfort," Joy recalled. "But he refused to talk to them about his own feelings."

"Many people say things to sick people just to make themselves feel better, which I consider to be the ultimate selfishness," Gary explained.

Gary's openness about his drug and criminal past made me risk asking another sensitive question. Gary and Joy were among the 600,000 people who participated in a national march on Washington in support of lesbian and gay rights. They even asked many of their straight friends to join them. I remarked that Gary seemed amazingly comfortable often being the only straight man in a roomful of gay men and lesbians. I asked him if he'd always been so comfortable around gay people.

"I didn't become 'nonhomophobic' when I got AIDS," Gary answered.

Joy jumped in: "Gary and I went to grade school together, so I've known him a long time. All his life, Gary was very different from everybody. He was one of those people who really didn't fit into any group, but who could get along with anybody. He had a painful childhood and a difficult family situation. I mean, he comes from a Jewish, middle-class background, and you might wonder, 'Well, how did someone like that become a heroin addict with a felony record?' But he's had a long history of major clashes that way. Gary always had the ability to blend in to all different situations. I mean, he's a New York, middle-class Jew who happens to be very intelligent, and he went to high school with a bunch of rednecks from Texas and lived all over the place. He's already crossed a lot of boundaries. This isn't the first one or the biggest one, or the greatest example of it. And that's what makes Gary very unusual. Because he has a strong sense of himself which allows him to not be threatened by other people's differences. And I think it's a really good thing and a positive strength in someone, but paradoxically it came from a sad and difficult experience of someone who always felt like an outsider."

Gary admitted that sometimes he was uncomfortable with the sexual banter that often takes place at Coalition board meetings, but concluded, "The fight that we are all involved in is so much more important than any differences. One thing that this crisis has shown me is how separate and ghettoized society makes us. I have met many, many wonderful, loving people as a result of these horrible circumstances, and a majority of them are gay. Except for this AIDS crisis, I'm sure I would never have met them, because the culture is so good at separating us."

"It's very hard being different," Joy observed. "The gay community has given us a lot of support and opened their arms totally to us, and we're very, very thankful for that. I think activism has been good for Gary and for me, but it's very isolating in other ways. Most of our friends are straight, and they are not involved in the AIDS community the way gay people are. We came back from that march feeling such a rush, and in turn we felt kind of alienated from our straight friends for a while."

Joy's love for Gary was palpable. It was clear that she would do whatever she had to to support Gary in his struggle against AIDS. She was even willing to explore macrobiotics with him briefly. "But it was very hard," Joy said. "I'm *addicted* to garlic."

"The simplest macrobiotic meals required tremendous preparation," Gary recalled. "And it became the same issue that I had had with AZT, actually: 'Am I going to do this in a committed way or am I not?' Now, I've compromised; I try to eat as healthfully as possible, but I'm not macrobiotic. I feel macrobiotics is a good thing for people early on, but not after you've gotten really sick. Then you need to put *on* weight, and the macrobiotic diet isn't good for gaining weight."

Gary had also dabbled with other holistic approaches to healing. "I think that there is a great deal of benefit that can be derived through herbal, holistic, or macrobiotic approaches. If that's what makes someone feel good, that's what they should be doing. I have gotten shiatsu massages and I tried acupuncture with Dr. Rabinowitz for a while when I had crypto. But we both agreed after a while that it wasn't working, so I stopped.

"But I also think that people who absolutely refuse to take any medicine are making a mistake. And holistic practitioners who strictly forbid people from taking medicine are doing a disservice to their patients. I think you can do both. I am a firm believer in self-empowerment and taking control of your own healing. But that very often crosses a very thin line of self-blame, you know? If you don't get better, does that mean you're not trying hard enough? That you're a failure?"

As my final question, I asked him what advice he would give to someone newly diagnosed.

"Have Don Kotler as your doctor," he said, without skipping a beat. "And get involved with the PWA Coalition." He elaborated: "I would try and impress upon them that they don't need to feel alone. A lot of people have gone through, and are going through, what they will go through, and these people can be there for you. Oh, and I'd tell them that AIDS is not a death sentence. I'd tell them to get good health care and to be aggressive about it. And whatever they do, they should make sure that they are an equal partner in making treatment choices. Don't be passive!

"And most importantly, people who've just been diagnosed should realize that AIDS is a *virus,* not something they deserve or something they caused to happen. I feel *very* strongly about this," he said.

3

LIFE IN
HELL

HOW LONG WILL YOU LIVE?

A FUN TEST

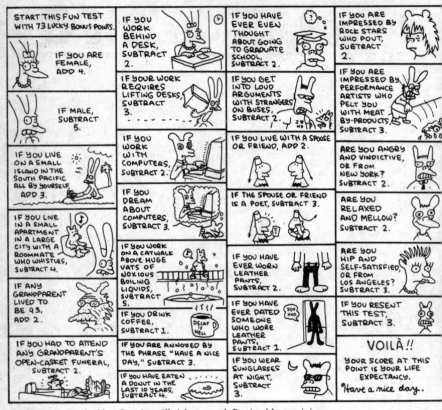

START THIS FUN TEST WITH 73 LUCKY BONUS POINTS.

IF YOU ARE FEMALE, ADD 4.

IF MALE, SUBTRACT 5.

IF YOU LIVE ON A SMALL ISLAND IN THE SOUTH PACIFIC ALL BY YOURSELF, ADD 3.

IF YOU LIVE IN A SMALL APARTMENT IN A LARGE CITY WITH A ROOMMATE WHO WHISTLES, SUBTRACT 4.

IF ANY GRANDPARENT LIVED TO BE 93, ADD 2.

IF YOU HAD TO ATTEND ANY GRANDPARENT'S OPEN-CASKET FUNERAL, SUBTRACT 2.

IF YOU WORK BEHIND A DESK, SUBTRACT 2.

IF YOUR WORK REQUIRES LIFTING DESKS, SUBTRACT 3.

IF YOU WORK WITH COMPUTERS, SUBTRACT 2.

IF YOU DREAM ABOUT COMPUTERS, SUBTRACT 3.

IF YOU WORK ON A CATWALK ABOVE HUGE VATS OF NOXIOUS BOILING LIQUIDS, SUBTRACT 5.

IF YOU DRINK COFFEE, SUBTRACT 1.

DECAF OF HELL

IF YOU ARE ANNOYED BY THE PHRASE "HAVE A NICE DAY," SUBTRACT 3.

IF YOU HAVE EATEN A DONUT IN THE LAST 10 YEARS, SUBTRACT 4.

IF YOU HAVE EVER EVEN THOUGHT ABOUT GOING TO GRADUATE SCHOOL, SUBTRACT 2.

IF YOU GET INTO LOUD ARGUMENTS WITH STRANGERS ON BUSES, SUBTRACT 2.

IF YOU LIVE WITH A SPOUSE OR FRIEND, ADD 2.

IF THE SPOUSE OR FRIEND IS A POET, SUBTRACT 3.

IF YOU HAVE EVER WORN LEATHER PANTS, SUBTRACT 2.

IF YOU HAVE EVER DATED SOMEONE WHO WORE LEATHER PANTS, SUBTRACT 1.

YOO HOO!

IF YOU WEAR SUNGLASSES AT NIGHT, SUBTRACT 3.

IF YOU ARE IMPRESSED BY ROCK STARS WHO POUT, SUBTRACT 2.

IF YOU ARE IMPRESSED BY PERFORMANCE ARTISTS WHO PELT YOU WITH MEAT BY-PRODUCTS, SUBTRACT 3.

ARE YOU ANGRY AND VINDICTIVE, OR FROM NEW YORK? SUBTRACT 2.

ARE YOU RELAXED AND MELLOW? SUBTRACT 2.

ARE YOU HIP AND SELF-SATISFIED, OR FROM LOS ANGELES? SUBTRACT 3.

IF YOU RESENT THIS TEST, SUBTRACT 3.

VOILÀ!!

YOUR SCORE AT THIS POINT IS YOUR LIFE EXPECTANCY.

Have a nice day.

MAKING SENSE OF SURVIVAL

▨▨▨ In addition to myself and the thirteen survivors profiled in this book, I have intensively interviewed a dozen more. I know casually, and know of, dozens of other long-term survivors. It seems that I know more long-term survivors than anyone in the world. It is both an honor and a burden.

The interviews and the research I've done make me feel that I have a pretty good sense of the factors that may contribute to long-term survival. My original suspicion has been confirmed: There are as many different ways to survive AIDS as there are survivors.

What stood out from the interviews was an ineffable quality of *joie de vivre*—a friskiness. These people didn't just believe that life was worth living—they all said in their own way that life was worth *celebrating*, and they were each busy doing precisely that. I can't say whether feeling incredibly grateful and glad to be alive is the cause, or the result, of having survived; probably, it's both.

If I had to describe in one word the characteristic common to all the survivors I interviewed, it would be *grit*. These people were all fighters: skeptical, opinionated, incredibly knowledgeable about AIDS, and passionately committed to living. They have worked hard to stay alive. They were all pragmatic optimists; they frequently reported that they had what is commonly referred to as "the right attitude," which basically meant that they had hope.

When I began interviewing long-term survivors, I had a secret fantasy. I imagined that I might inadvertently discover that all of them were doing something in common. I could then simply announce my miraculous finding to the world and the AIDS crisis would be over! Unfortunately, that didn't prove to be the case.

I had particularly hoped to discover that all survivors just happened to be using the same drugs. Because I'm a great believer in the importance of taking medication to prevent PCP, I had expected to find that all, or at least most, of the survivors were also taking medication to prevent the deadly pneumonia. I was wrong. At the time of most of the interviews (1987), few were on any form of PCP prophylaxis. However, most are now taking medication to prevent PCP.

In fact, survivors surprised me by expressing a generally cautious attitude toward experimental drugs. My sense is that such skepticism is a striking difference between old-timers and the newly diagnosed. It has been my experience that most newly diagnosed people with AIDS would sell their grandmothers for a crack at getting the hot experimental drug-of-the-month. Often, the recently diagnosed are frantic to do *something*— take some pill—and are willing to risk extraordinary toxicity for the usually hollow promise of extending their lives even a couple of months. Having survived beyond predictions seems to allow the luxury of thinking about the long term, which leads survivors to be skeptical—at times, even cynical—about the experimental-drug roller coaster.

Although several survivors had entered experimental treatment protocols involving highly toxic drugs, most had quickly abandoned them or drastically reduced the dosages—often without the knowledge or consent of their physician. Survivors had watched too many friends suffer the agonies of complications of toxic experimental drugs only to die anyway. The common wisdom shared among most survivors was that as long as one was stable, the risks of experimental drugs often outweighed the potential benefits.

To my shock and delight, this skepticism about drugs extended even to the use of AZT. I've kept in touch with most of the survivors whom I interviewed (including those whose profiles aren't in this book). As of spring 1990, only five of the long-term survivors profiled here (and only one of the dozen who aren't included) had ever tried AZT—despite unbelievably intense pressure to do so. Three of the five profiled who had taken AZT did so very reluctantly and for a very short time and had abandoned it entirely at the first sign of toxicity. When pressed to explain why they hadn't hopped on the AZT bandwagon, most echoed some version of "If it ain't broke, don't fix it." This didn't mean that they denied that they are immune-deficient. But I found an almost superstitious, don't-rock-the-boat attitude. It was as if, having made it this far, they were afraid to change anything for fear of jinxing their success. As John Lorenzini put it, he and his doctor believe in the doctrine of "DFWS: Don't fuck with success."

Since I had suffered tremendous abuse for my anti-AZT heresy, it was reassuring to discover that I am not alone in my belief that it is extremely unlikely that anyone will be a long-term survivor of AIDS if at the same time he or she attempts to be a long-term survivor of AZT.

All of the survivors had dabbled with what are generally referred to as holistic approaches to healing. While several reported that their physicians expressed skepticism about the benefits of a particular alternative approach, such skepticism never took the form of denigrating or forbidding the patient's choice. The attitude shared by physician and patient was that if something may help and can't hurt, why not try it? Neither doctor nor patient underestimated the importance of palliative interventions. As one survivor put it, "Ultimately, the best indication of how you feel is, well . . . how you feel. And if, say, I find that acupuncture reduces the side effects of chemotherapy, or if a particular diet makes me feel like I have more energy, why not stick with it, without demanding to know how or why it works?"

Only one long-term survivor, Roberto, has completely turned his back on Western medicine in favor of macrobiotics, and he positively glows with health. This proves that Western medicine, with all its powerful, often toxic drugs, is not the only way to survive AIDS.

The fact that virtually every survivor (including me) has explored various holistic approaches to AIDS fascinated me. But as was the case with allopathic drugs, no single holistic therapy was common to all.

Most survivors said that *before* AIDS, they would never have considered holistics—although a significant minority of survivors had been vaguely New Age prior to diagnosis (particularly the California contingent).

My explanation for the sudden interest in holistics is this: Since science and medicine have failed utterly to provide any certainty in the realm of treatments, it makes sense to remain open-minded about other therapies. Aside from AZT, there are no FDA-approved therapies for the underlying immunodeficiency of AIDS. Survivors felt they had nothing to lose by modifying the standards of "proof" required.

Openness to holistics was indicative of a more general open-mindedness. The willingness to consider "unproven," nontraditional healing approaches requires a leap of faith more characteristic of spirituality than of the rationalism of the scientific method. Not surprisingly, perhaps, a sudden interest in spirituality and religion was another pattern that emerged. A majority of the survivors spoke of returning to the faiths of their childhood and to attending church regularly. They found great comfort in thinking about a loving god/dess and life after death.

Frankly, I was nauseated by all the talk of God and similar higher powers. Religious sentiment certainly hasn't played *any* role in my own survival—at least not so far as I can tell. I say "at least not so far as I can tell" because I recently discovered that my Methodist mother has organized a prayer group that regularly prays for my healing. When she told me about it, I was simultaneously deeply moved and horrified. I have no use for religion, but I recognized that this was my mother's way of showing her love and concern.

Could prayer actually be healing? The idea seems ludicrous to me, but while researching the literature on psychoneuroimmunology, I came across a fascinating double-blind study that found that a group of people who had had surgery and whose names had been given to a prayer circle without their knowledge had a significantly lower incidence of post-op complications and death than did a matched group of people who weren't prayed for. The fact that none of the surgery subjects knew they were being prayed for rules out the possibility of a placebo effect. Perhaps humans communicate concern for each other in ways not yet understood.

But when I begin to seriously entertain such metaphysical mush, my rational mind balks. The idea that I'm alive because a well-meaning group of Midwestern housewives include me in their prayers just makes no sense to someone as rabidly, rigidly rational as I am. I'm more comfortable just calling it luck—the atheist's noun of choice to explain the unexplainable.

I resist some survivors' assertions that credit for their hard-won survival belongs to a higher power. It seemed to me that these people had done extraordinarily difficult work, swimming upstream against powerful currents of skepticism and fatalism. I felt they ought to take more of the credit for themselves, rather than giving credit to some obscure force from beyond. Their stories made it clear that they worked hard to stay alive—so hard, in fact, that the friend of one survivor who was doing well chided him: "You should go off disability and get a full-time job." The survivor retorted: "I have a full-time job: surviving AIDS." He then recounted that day's grueling schedule, which involved acupuncture, visualization, shopping for organic food, attending support groups, participating in an experimental-drug trial, and attending an AIDS political demonstration.

My explanation for the recrudescence of religious sentiment among long-term survivors would be this: We need hope to survive. And when rational systems offer no hope, we turn to those systems that do. In our culture, that means religious systems that speak of life after death, of meaning to suffering, of a caring god (or goddess) who will take care of you.

Finally, nearly all of the survivors were involved to some extent in the politics of AIDS. Some have publicly identified themselves as people with AIDS, and some even as long-term survivors—both courageous, political acts that often lead to discrimination and hostility. Others' political involvement was quieter and more personal, like starting or actively participating in PWA support groups, often long after they themselves had stopped drawing much benefit from attending them.

It may well be that politics is an antidote to the self-obsession that can accompany AIDS. To realize that there's someone worse off, whom you can help, can be an incredible relief—and maybe even healing.

⊠ How does the profile of AIDS survivors proposed by the psychoneuroimmunologists hold up based on the interviews I did?

The problem I have with many of the hypotheses about long-term AIDS survivors developed by Dr. Solomon and Dr. Temoshok is that, like horoscopes, they are often hopelessly general. "Characteristics" and "emotional states" are slippery and subjective concepts. Psychometric techniques that attempt to measure such elusive states as "hopelessness" or "helplessness" or "hardiness" seem scientifically suspect to me.

Still, by and large, Drs. Solomon and Temoshok have captured the essence of the survivors I interviewed.

As they predicted, survivors were realistic about the seriousness of their condition. But I'm not sure it's fair to say that survivors were never fatalistic. In fact, every survivor spoke of despairing at times. The most frequent strategy was to ignore—rather than to deny—the fatalistic propaganda.

As Solomon and Temoshok predicted, the survivors I interviewed took responsibility for their own healing, and this expressed itself in a number of ways. Many voiced strong opinions about the need to acknowledge some personal responsibility for life-style choices, both in terms of getting sick in the first place and in terms of getting well. However, several were quick to carefully distinguish the notion of taking responsibility for getting well from the counterproductive attitude of blaming oneself for being sick.

Taking personal responsibility for healing meant making difficult and major life-style changes. With the exception of Emilio (who continued to drink heavily) and Cristofer (who continued to abuse drugs for several years after his diagnosis and didn't make major changes until after he'd become a long-term survivor), all the survivors profoundly curtailed their use of recreational drugs and alcohol soon after diagnosis. Most also went through a period of radical diet change, although with the exception of Roberto, everyone eventually reverted to old eating habits. All the gay survivors had radically altered their sex lives and had either become celibate or made the difficult adjustment to safe sex.

Another expression of taking responsibility for healing took the form of listening to their own bodies—staying attuned to the messages that the body sends. Survivors observed that prior to diagnosis, they had often pushed their bodies beyond endurance and had willfully ignored warning signals. Now, because they recognized that AIDS might kill them, they gave themselves permission to be more responsive to the messages their bodies might be sending. They were willing to nurture, even pamper, themselves.

Taking responsibility for healing also meant a willingness to resolve conflict in their lives. Most quit stressful jobs and began pursuing activities that gave them pleasure. Many also made it a priority to resolve emotional conflict by weeding out friends, family, and lovers who were not supportive.

One characteristic of survivors proposed by Solomon and Temoshok that wasn't borne out by my interviews concerned exercise. As someone who never knowingly embarks on any course of action that might, even accidentally, lead to physical exertion or, god forbid, sweating, I can assert that exercise has played absolutely no role in my own survival. The survivors who exercise regularly were a distinct minority.

Also, none of the survivors articulated any "unmet goals" of a grand nature; none said that they only wanted to live long enough to write the great American novel, or make a million dollars, or settle the Middle East conflict. Goals tended to be more modest—like making it through one more day.

As predicted by the psychoneuroimmunologic portrait of PWA long-term survivors, most could be described as assertive and able to say no. But again, whether they are more so than PWAs who don't survive is an unanswered question. I certainly have known PWAs who were just as feisty and empowered as some of these survivors but who nevertheless succumbed to AIDS. They went down *fighting*, but they went down.

⊠ Meeting other survivors made it very clear to me that attitude matters. The human mind is a great, largely untapped pharmacy, and it behooves anyone facing a life-threatening illness to investigate ways to harness this tremendous resource.

It simply makes sense to try to mobilize whatever immune-enhancing effects might flow from marshaling the mind. After all, even if your

T-cells don't increase, how can having a cheerful, frisky, life-affirming attitude possibly hurt?

On the other hand, I'm troubled by those who believe that attitude is all—that the search for drugs isn't really necessary because if only you love yourself enough, you can *will* AIDS away. This seems to me to be a dangerous oversimplification of available evidence.

The most I'm willing to say is that having the right attitude (which I define as loving and nurturing yourself, loving life enough to fight for it, and believing that surviving AIDS is possible) is the necessary precondition for long-term survival. Having the right attitude won't guarantee that you'll survive AIDS, but the inverse appears to be true: Being fatalistic and losing your will to live pretty much guarantees that you'll die swiftly from AIDS.

I am convinced by the interviews that there is a "will to live"—that all humans harbor a survival instinct. But it seems that to survive AIDS, this survival instinct—this will to live—must be aggressively encouraged.

Sometimes I'm too rational for my own good. Most of the long-term survivors I interviewed seemed completely disinterested in survival probabilities and possible scientific explanations for their own survival. They often preferred to take leaps of faith into the blind alleys of alternative and allopathic approaches to AIDS. I envied their ability to suspend disbelief and do what made them feel good without first insisting on a detailed, referenced, rational explanation for precisely *how* a particular treatment approach was supposed to work. But my inquiring mind simply *had* to know why and how. Even a rationalist can see the advantages to being assertive, doing an emotional housecleaning, and loving life. Whether, and precisely how, such characteristics and behaviors actually contribute to longevity are open questions; but they undoubtedly improve the *quality* of life and for that reason alone can be recommended for everyone.

In the absence of a magic bullet, there simply is no one way to survive AIDS. Every survivor expressed the sentiment that each person with AIDS would have to follow his or her own instincts and trust his or her own judgment.

WHAT I WOULD DO
IF I WERE YOU

▨▨▨ For the last two years, I have traveled the country talking to people with AIDS about long-term survival. People always ask me what I think *they* should do, particularly which drugs they should take. Aside from urging everyone with AIDS to take medication to prevent PCP, I have resisted giving detailed advice. I didn't want my biases to unduly influence others' life-and-death choices. But because the different perspectives of many survivors have been included in this book, I feel more comfortable speaking my mind.

So, for the hundreds who have asked, here, for the first (and last) time, is what I would do if I were you.

1. Decide if you really want to live.

Soon after being diagnosed, you will have to go off by yourself to some quiet place and ask some hard questions. First and foremost, do you really want to live? Are you willing to draw on every reserve of strength that you possess in order to put up the fight of your life?

I know it's offensive to suggest that some people don't want to live, but many survivors talked about the temptation to just check out—end the struggle. I've known people with AIDS who felt that they never controlled their own lives. They often react to their AIDS diagnosis with a strange sense of relief, a calm resignation. *At last* there is some certainty in their lives; they are almost relieved to know how the story is going to end. Such people shut down emotionally and give in to the conveyor-belt conceptualization of AIDS. They lose the will to live and, with it, the will to fight. Death usually follows swiftly, like the self-fulfilling prophecy it has become.

Often, this doomed, helpless attitude isn't conscious. Sometimes it gets expressed by a sigh from deep in the soul or a quiet shrug of the shoulders that says, "I don't really care whether I live or die." But I have never seen anyone who has lost the will to fight to survive AIDS. Long-term survivors are very clear about wanting to squeeze the last possible drop out of life. The only way to beat such a formidable foe as AIDS is to love life *fiercely*. You have to make a conscious choice that life is precious and that you want to enjoy it for as long as possible. And it helps to have a clear image of yourself as a survivor.

The will to live is a mysterious but powerful force. You've simply got to have it to survive.

2. Spring clean emotionally.

AIDS can either be viewed as a sign to begin dying or as a challenge to begin living. Use AIDS as a catalyst for making the changes you've been putting off all of your life. AIDS is a challenge to become who you've always wanted to be. Give yourself permission to make any difficult changes you've been putting off.

Put on your babushka, get out that feather duster, and roll up your sleeves; it's time for some emotional housecleaning. Surround yourselves with those who love you and those whom you love. Where possible, make peace and resolve conflict. Where that's not possible, cut bait and move on.

AIDS makes you realize how insignificant and petty most conflict is.

Being diagnosed with AIDS can be like going through ten years of therapy in a weekend. It's a crash course in assertiveness. If you can't ask for what you need now, you may never get another chance. Seize the opportunity to be truly happy.

3. Fall in love.

I highly recommend falling in love if you haven't done so lately. If you choose the right mate(s), loving and being loved can be quite healing.

Don't for a second think AIDS is an excuse to give up on love. At the lowest moment of my life—the week I was officially diagnosed—I met the man of my dreams. He was wonderful enough, or crazy enough, to gamble on loving somebody everyone told him would be dead in six months. If he'd listened to the naysayers, or if I had clung to my belief that I was factory seconds/damaged merchandise, we'd both have missed out on the last eight wonderful years together. Make no mistake about it: Life and love after diagnosis are definite possibilities.

For terminally shy PWAs, many PWA Coalitions conduct singles' teas that provide a low-pressure setting for people with AIDS (and those who wish to date us) to meet and mate. (I myself have become a yenta; I have fixed up many people and currently have a whole stable of eligible PWA bachelors and bachelorettes, straight, gay, bisexual, and lesbian. The fee for my services: your firstborn.)

4. Decide whether participating in support groups with others will be helpful or depressing, and act accordingly.

Sharing survival strategies with other people with AIDS can be invaluable. Plugging into the PWA network gives you access to the latest treatment news, often long before it appears anywhere else. People who are going through the same thing as you often have a wealth of practical information that can make your journey easier. I strongly recommend that everyone diagnosed join a support group. And I recommend that you make a commitment to attend at least three meetings, just to give it a fair chance. On the other hand, don't stick with a group that isn't meeting your needs. Shop around.

Some people eventually find support groups tedious or depressing. Their strategy is to lead as normal a life as possible and to avoid becoming a professional PWA. It works for some. Do whatever works for you.

5. Decide who, if anyone, you want to tell about your diagnosis.

Generally, full disclosure is best. It's too stressful to try to remember who knows and who doesn't. And often, as is the case with coming out as a gay person, once you do, you realize that everybody knew all along anyway.

But AIDS discrimination is real and can be devastating, and not every PWA has the stamina to endure it. There's no rule. Just realize that once you tell a single person, there's no turning back. A secret as juicy as an AIDS diagnosis usually cannot be kept by even the most well-intentioned friend or loved one.

6. Set reasonable, achievable goals for yourself.

One day at a time is how you become a long-term survivor. By concentrating on the quality of each day, you may wake up years from now to discover that you've lived a very long time. Don't set unreasonable goals that you aren't likely to be able to achieve and then use your failure to achieve them as an excuse to beat up on yourself. Don't, for example, say, I'm going to will my lesions away and they'll all be gone by this time next week! Be patient and give yourself credit for the small, incremental improvements that each day brings.

This is not to say that long-term goals are out of the question. For example, if going back to college is something you've always wanted to do, do it. Don't hesitate just because some asshole tells you that your chances of finishing four years are slim. I know several PWAs who went back to school after they were diagnosed who recently received their degrees.

7. Get political.

All the long-term survivors I've interviewed have been involved to some extent in the political struggle surrounding AIDS. Being political has several potential advantages: It may actually change the world and make it a better place for yourself and for others; it can help you keep your own problems in perspective; and, if the psychoneuroimmunoligists are right, protesting and marching and shouting helps you get rid of all that nasty, immunosuppressive anger and frustration.

8. Prepare for the worst, and then hope for the best.

Although certain forms of denial have their uses, it's not a good idea to ignore the real possibility that you may die sooner rather than later. Facing the prospect of your own death squarely has the paradoxical effect of freeing you to get on with the business of living.

Be practical. Make contact with individuals and organizations knowledgeable about AIDS. There are many resources available to you that you never imagined. Make sure your insurance is paid up. Find the right doctor. Make a will. Give someone power of attorney to make medical decisions for you in the event that you can't. Communicate to your doctor and your loved ones how you feel about pain management and extraordinary life-support measures. While you're lucid and calm, make sure those around you understand—and will respect—your decisions.

Decide how and under what circumstances you want to die. (I, for one, intend to die the old-fashioned way: at home, in my own bed, surrounded by those I love.) Then, once you've prepared for death, forget about it. Turn your attention to the formidable task of staying alive and living life to its fullest. Be hopeful and optimistic—even cheerful. Surround yourselves with others who support your hope. Avoid those who patronize you, or hand you *On Death and Dying* every time you mention that you intend to survive AIDS.

I don't want to be glib. I know it's hard to sustain hope when you're feeling like shit. I too am often nauseated by the "Church of the Happy Face" and by the New Age gurus who imply that all you have to do to survive AIDS is love yourself. I recoil from the implication of such simplistic metaphysics that anyone who dies must not have loved him- or herself enough. But the New Agers are right about one thing: If you're going to find the strength and endurance you'll need to wrestle this beast to the ground, you'll have to love yourself.

I highly recommend daily doses of laughter, nature, beauty, and art. Loving and being loved feed and sustain hope and are very healing. Do anything and everything that reaffirms the preciousness of life, and then live each moment—each day—to the fullest.

9. Follow your grandmother's advice: all things in moderation.

Use plain ol' common sense. Eat nutritious food. Then eat some more. Get plenty of sleep. Don't abuse your body with drugs and alcohol. Practice safer sex. Without being paranoid about it, try to avoid other diseases. Reduce the distress in your life. Quit a job that you hate. Do more of the things that give you pleasure and less of the things that stress you out. Then call your grandmother and give her the thrill of hearing you tell her that she was right all along.

10. Doubt all things, beginning with the advice in this book. Cultivate an attitude of appropriate skepticism, of radical doubt. Seek out diverse viewpoints.

"At least once in your life, doubt all things," advised eighteenth-century scientist and philosopher René Descartes. Great advice, especially when your life is at stake. Skepticism doesn't require believing that everyone is out to get you. More often, it's perfectly well-intentioned people whose mistakes can cost you your life. Don't die of politeness. Don't be afraid that questioning someone's advice may hurt their feelings. *Not* questioning it may hurt *you.* It may even kill you.

Twentieth-century humanist Erich Fromm had a useful definition of radical doubt that is perfectly applicable to AIDS:

> By radicalism, I do not refer primarily to a certain set of ideas, but rather to an attitude, to an "approach," as it were. To begin with, this approach can be characterized by the motto: *de omnibus dubitandum;* everything must be doubted, particularly the ideological concepts which are shared by virtually everybody and have consequently assumed the role of indubitable commonsensical axioms. To "doubt" in this sense . . . [implies] the readiness and capacity for critical questioning of all assumptions and institutions which have become idols under the name common sense, logic, and what is supposed to be "natural."[1]

Radical doubt doesn't have to be stridently expressed. In fact, you'll often get more mileage out of being polite but persistent. Express your genuine curiosity rather than implying that someone is trying to put something over on you.

Far too many people with AIDS want to be told what to do. Options only confuse them; they don't like to take responsibility for making decisions. Although there may be people who've survived AIDS by putting blind faith in their doctors, I've not met them.

People who are seriously committed to helping you save your life will understand your questioning. They will understand that you are searching for the truth, and that truth benefits from being tested by skepticism. The best doctors encourage their patients to share responsibility for healing.

Experts disagree about what is causing AIDS and how best to treat it. Seeking out diverse views will allow you to make choices that are truly informed. Unfortunately, it's human nature to first decide what one thinks is true, and then go in search of supporting evidence. Any fact that complicates or contradicts one's original view is then ignored or rejected. It's vital that people with AIDS fight this natural tendency.

Scientific or medical truth cannot be determined in a democratic fashion. The fact that a majority agrees that something is true is certainly worth noting, but it doesn't mean you can afford not to find out why the minority rejects that view. The minority may, after all, be right.

If Dr. A tells you to ignore Dr. B's advice, ask why. If Dr. A says it's because Dr. B is "wacko," that's often a sign that Dr. A is unable to refute the "wacko's" assertions. Those who resort to below-the-belt *ad hominem* attacks are often trying to cover up the fact that they can't really defend their views.

Sometimes "crazy" people say the sanest things, and when you have AIDS, you ignore differing viewpoints at your peril. The history of scientific controversy is replete with instances where heretics who spoke out against the commonsensical wisdom of the day were excommunicated, burned at the stake, tortured, ruined financially, or driven insane for saying things that were subsequently proven to be true. That's why it's so important to judge a viewpoint on its merits and not by how its proponents dress or where they went to school.

11. **Do your homework. Educate yourself about AIDS and your body.**
Now is not the time to be lazy or passive. Read as much about AIDS and the immune system and drugs as you can stomach. There are hundreds of AIDS newsletters, books, and tapes; use them.

Don't be overawed by credentials or titles. Pay more attention to track record. Is the person giving advice right more often than she or he is wrong?

Familiarize yourself with drugs and their potential side effects. Learn to read the *Physicians' Desk Reference (PDR),* which lists known side effects of drugs. Be on the lookout for signs of adverse drug interactions. No one else—not even your doctor—can look out for your interests better than you can. Looking out for yourself will require that you understand your body, your disease, and your options.

12. Trust your instincts and your common sense.

One of the most important lessons I've learned from AIDS was taught to me by my doctor. By patiently answering, in simple language, all my questions about how the immune system works and what drugs do, he has shown me that anyone can be made to understand anything if the person explaining it truly *wants* the other person to understand.

Most medical doctors tend to use highly technical language, even when they don't have to. This often has the effect of intimidating patients into not asking questions, out of the mistaken belief that they couldn't possibly understand what the doctor is talking about. Nonsense! Insist that your physician speak in plain English (or whatever language you prefer). Persist. Say, "I'm sorry. I don't understand. Could you please explain it again?"

It's *your* body that will benefit or suffer from a doctor's recommendation. Love yourself enough to ask as many questions as you need to have answered to make an informed decision.

13. Choose the right doctor(s) and begin negotiating a healing partnership.

I often joke that physicians are like stereos—they'll all play your records; it's just a question of what your ears like. It's amazing how many people with AIDS are unhappy with their doctors but are unwilling, or unable, to switch.

The doctor/patient relationship is one of the most intimate relationships humans can form: Your physician pokes and prods you, sticks things inside you, and subjects you to painful, potentially dangerous procedures. You literally trust him or her with your life.

Before you enter a relationship of such profound intimacy and importance, you should make a list of the characteristics you'd like in a doctor. For example, he or she should: have experience caring for people with AIDS; be willing to spend as much time with you as you need; be willing to answer your questions in terms you can understand; understand and share your world view regarding drugs, pain management, and death; have admitting privileges at the hospital you prefer; welcome the idea of a healing partnership. Once you've made your list, shop around and hold out for what you want.

To double-check that you're making the right choice, plug into the

PWA grapevine and identify other patients of the physician you've chosen. Ask them about their experience with this doctor.

Another quick test of whether the physician you've chosen is the right one for you is to ask him or her how he or she would feel if you sought out a second opinion. A competent, self-assured physician should welcome it rather than be threatened by it. Ask how he or she will feel when you bring medical literature to his or her attention. Make sure he or she is open-minded about alternative therapies. Ask your doctor to explain what he or she thinks is causing AIDS, because it will affect how he or she approaches treatment. Steer clear of those doctors who ignore or downplay toxicity in a belief that HIV must be stopped at any price. After all, you're the one who will have to endure the neuropathy and rash and fevers and other horrific side effects that might result from having made the wrong choice about an experimental drug.

Finally, ask your prospective physician how long a patient with AIDS is likely to survive. If he or she gives grim, dire predictions and communicates hopelessness, then that has probably been his or her experience. This would suggest that he or she doesn't understand that how aggressively a doctor manages his or her patient will play a major role in how long that patient lives, or that he or she may have become burnt out by all the death and suffering. Find a doctor who is optimistic and who will support your own optimism.

14. Prophylax against opportunistic infections.

PWAs die from a number of well-recognized diseases, many of which are preventable. Talk with your doctor about the concept of prophylaxis in general, and about PCP prophylaxis in particular. Does he or she think you should start taking low doses of antifungal medication to prevent thrush and cryptococcal meningitis? If you have antibodies to toxoplasmosis, would he or she prescribe pyrimethamine and leucovorin, even though proper clinical trials have not been completed? What about high-dose acyclovir to control herpes virus reactivations? Your physician must understand the importance of prophylaxis for all the major opportunistic infections. Make sure he or she is willing to at least consider trying relatively nontoxic ways to prevent lethal diseases without insisting on proof from a placebo-controlled trial.

15. When considering what drugs to take, concentrate first on those that may or may not help but that probably won't hurt.

Exhaust all nontoxic, or less toxic, treatment options before resorting to highly toxic therapies.

I've frankly never understood why some people prefer to start with drugs known to be incredibly toxic. A healthy, asymptomatic HIV-seropositive person taking AZT is like someone who detonates a thermonuclear warhead to rid his or her home of cockroaches. The warhead may (or may not) bring your roach problem under control, but at the cost of eliminating you and your house along with it.

Although it's heresy to say so, sometimes doing nothing is better than doing something that may harm you. The peer pressure to take highly toxic drugs like AZT and ddI (dideoxyinosine) is enormous, but don't give in just because someone badgers you into it.

16. Don't take AZT.

Surviving AIDS is hard enough without attempting, at the same time, to survive AZT's toxicity. AZT and similar nucleoside analogues were abandoned by researchers years ago as *unfit for human use.* It's curious that AZT was pulled off the shelf to be given to gays and IV drug users.

AZT is what is known as a DNA-chain terminator. (Just think of it as "The Terminator" for short.) My doctor has succinctly stated that in the long term, "AZT is incompatible with life," because DNA synthesis is the basis of all life.

AZT is also carcinogenic. It kills cells and prevents your body from generating new ones. Must I go on?

Add impotence to the list of horrendous side effects. No, you won't find impotence listed as a side effect in the 1987/88 PDR—a fact that one PWA who developed impotence after a year of full-dose AZT intends to use as the basis of a lawsuit against Burroughs Wellcome. Don't let anyone fool you into believing that impotence is a common complication of AIDS itself. Anecdotal evidence suggests that the promiscuous prescribing of AZT is resulting in chemical castration of "undesirable" populations.

I realize that many people with AIDS reading this book are taking AZT. All I can say is: Less is more and none is best. Why not consider going to half-dose or even quarter-dose? Why not combine it with high-dose acyclovir and low-dose naltrexone? Better yet, why not do acyclovir and naltrexone instead? Certainly skip your nighttime dose; your sleep will do you more good than AZT.

If you insist on taking AZT or its toxic cousin, ddI, be sure to monitor your blood regularly for signs of toxicity. (Anemia is the most common side effect; the "droopy butt" syndrome caused by muscle wasting is also common.) Reduce the dose or stop altogether at the first sign of toxicity. Maybe by the time this book is published, the community-based research movement will have begun testing a multimodal approach to AIDS that doesn't involve such toxic drugs. Keep up-to-date about alternatives to AZT.

17. Avoid federally designed clinical trials.

The federal government's track record of unethical, poorly designed trials speaks for itself. Unless there are major changes in the design and execution of government AIDS trials, approach them with extreme caution.

If you have 200 or fewer T-helper cells, never enter a clinical trial that forbids PCP prophylaxis. Don't be willing to die for the supposed greater good of the greater numbers. Besides, a government trial is likely to be so poorly designed and executed that the data will end up being worthless anyway.

If you're desperate to enter a clinical trial, check out the community-based research groups in your area. At least there you or your representatives can have some input into the design of the trial.

18. Make peace with uncertainty and contradiction. Admit that you will have to make treatment decisions on the basis of inconclusive evidence.

One often hears these days that AIDS has somehow suddenly become a chronic, manageable disease. This suggests that the crisis is over and that all a PWA has to do is subscribe to a few treatment newsletters to be let in on the big secret of how to survive AIDS. I wish somebody would tell *me* what treatments, aside from AZT, are supposed to produce this remarkable result. Where is the data to support this claim?

The truth is we will never know with any certainty which drugs work and which don't until we bite the bullet and do properly conducted clinical trials. In the meantime, every person with AIDS has to make peace with the fact that s/he will be forced to make difficult treatment choices on the basis of confusing and conflicting evidence.

There are many substances that PWAs are injecting, ingesting, and imbibing. Some of these drugs may actually be slowing the progression of AIDS. But because we haven't done the research to prove it, we may never know and the chaos will continue.

There are three kinds of evidence on which it is reasonable to make treatment decisions:

    a. *Firsthand reports from individuals who've tried particular therapies.*
       Obviously, anecdotal reports are not conclusive. Just because someone trashes a drug that didn't work for him/her doesn't mean it won't work for you. Conversely, just because someone swears that a substance or therapy saved his or her life doesn't mean it will have the same effect on you. Each of us is genetically and biochemically different and so we respond to interventions differently.

       Obviously, the more people who've tried a particular approach and had the same result, the more you are justified in having confidence in what they say.

b. *Theoretical evidence.*

Often, a strong case can be made for trying a particular approach with AIDS on the basis of its success in treating a similar disease. For example, it is generally agreed that the herpes family of viruses plays a role in accelerating the progression of AIDS. Each of the six herpes viruses share similar mechanisms of action. Acyclovir has been proven to be safe and effective in preventing the reactivation of herpes simplex types I and II. Although acyclovir is not yet approved as a therapy against any of the other herpes viruses, several researchers have noticed that people with AIDS who take lots of acyclovir tend not to have serious problems with any of the other herpes viruses. It therefore makes theoretical sense to me for people with AIDS to take high-dose acyclovir, since it may prevent the reactivation of CMV, EBV (Epstein-Barr virus), and shingles *and* it is relatively nontoxic. Thus, it is a drug that may or may not help slow the progression of AIDS but that is not likely to cause harm.

With AIDS, one doesn't have the luxury of waiting for definitive proof that a particular therapeutic approach works. It is reasonable, in the absence of proof, to act on the basis of a sound theoretical possibility that something might work, bearing in mind the potential for toxicity and harm.

c. *Data from a properly designed and conducted clinical trial.*

Many people mistakenly believe that all clinical trials are created equal. As the original inept AZT multicenter trial amply demonstrated, this is not the case. Before deciding to take a drug because you've been told that a clinical trial has "proven" that it works, read the actual report of the study and see if it makes sense to you. Talk to experts who might be aware of flaws in the design, execution, and analysis of the study.

19. Keep an open mind about holistic or alternative approaches to healing.

Western science has so far failed to find successful treatments for immune deficiency. One would think, therefore, that Western doctors would be a bit more humble than they are. Instead, they continue to arrogantly attack holistic therapies, as if they are more useless than the toxic allopathic drugs that have failed so miserably.

There is no question that holistic therapies can relieve symptoms. Symptom relief is no small achievement and only a fool would refuse to try something that will make him/her feel better just because Western medicine says it shouldn't work!

⊠ Every person's experience of AIDS will be unique. Tailor the preceding recommendations to fit your personality and your circumstances. Think of AIDS as a long-distance marathon. Pace yourself.

Remember: Anything is possible. Miracles happen. It's as reasonable to believe that you'll be lucky as it is to believe you are doomed. The worst that might happen is that you'll fail. But then again, you may live just long enough to be around for the cure that community-based research is going to find. Stick around for the celebration. It's gonna be some party!

NOTES

1. From Erich Fromm's Introduction to Illich, Ivan, *Celebration of Awareness*, New York: Heyday Books, 1970.

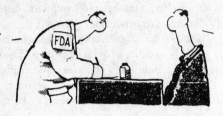

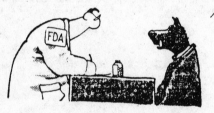

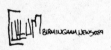

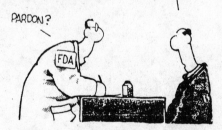

THE CASE AGAINST AZT

▨▨▨ AIDS is survivable without AZT.

I have survived AIDS for nearly eight years without popping a single AZT pill.

The overwhelming majority of long-term survivors I interviewed have eschewed AZT.

All of the 119 long-term survivors studied by the CDC survived AIDS before AZT was even available.

Since AZT wasn't available prior to 1985, the handful of people retrospectively diagnosed with AIDS back to 1978 and 1979 who are still alive today survived six or seven years without any AZT.[1]

Compare this with AZT's track record.

The last surviving patient from the original AZT trial, according to Burroughs Wellcome, died recently. When he died, he had been on AZT for three and one half years. He was the longest-surviving AZT recipient.[2]

AZT was first tested as a therapy for AIDS in 1985. Since its approval by the FDA as a treatment for AIDS in 1987, I have joined my doctor, Joe Sonnabend, and a handful of others in questioning the value of AZT. The debate over AZT—who should use it, at what dose, and when one should begin taking it—has been one of the most bitter and contentious of my AIDS career.

Those who are *convinced* that AZT extends life have accused AZT's critics of being complicit in the death of any PWA who was discouraged from trying AZT and who subsequently died. Even those who agree that AZT has probably been oversold and overprescribed nevertheless attack us for "stealing people's hope."

Recently, however, encouraging signs have appeared which suggest that more and more people are beginning to recognize that AZT may be doing more harm than good. Closeted AZT skeptics are beginning to fight back. According to an article[3] that appeared in the prestigious *Journal of the American Medical Association:*

> Scientists are not unanimous in endorsing . . . AZT . . . therapy for patients infected with the human immunodeficiency virus (HIV) whose CD4 cell counts are above 200/mm. Doubts are most notable among investigators at the Veterans Administration (VA) and in Europe who have not seen benefit in such patients in their own ongoing trials with the only approved drug that fights the retrovirus thought to cause acquired immunodeficiency syndrome (AIDS). . . . Skeptics point out that, according to the NIAID data, 100 patients must take zidovudine for a year to prevent four infections [infections, such as PCP] which for the most part can be . . . [prevented] . . . by other means. Everyone agrees that questions of long-term benefit, survival, toxicity, and resistance to the drug are unanswered. And some doubt the interpretation of temporarily increased CD4 counts as a benefit.

Further exciting evidence of a major sea change is a recent ad campaign attacking AZT, designed by Gran Fury, the artists collective responsible for the distinctive graphics of the AIDS Coalition to Unleash Power (ACT-UP).

The visually arresting ad uses the bold red-and-white design scheme of Coca-Cola ads but substitutes instead the phrase "Enjoy AZT." The text says:

> The U.S. government has spent one billion dollars over the past 10 years to research new AIDS drugs. The result? 1 drug—AZT. It makes half the people who try it sick and for the other half it stops working after a year. Is AZT the last, best hope for people with AIDS, or is it a short-cut to the killing Burroughs Wellcome is making in the AIDS marketplace? Scores of drugs languish in government pipelines, while fortunes are made on this monopoly. IS THIS HEALTH CARE OR WEALTH CARE?

While not a wholesale dismissal of AZT, the ad is evidence of a new desire to withdraw activist support for the use of AZT. The assertion that "AZT stops working after a year" implies that AZT works for a year in those PWAs who can tolerate it at all. While I challenge this assertion, the fact that a major ad campaign so critical of AZT is emanating from ACT-UP suggests that the truth about AZT may be widely admitted sooner than I had once thought possible.

▨ It has been more than four years since the first AZT clinical trial began. If AZT truly extended life, we'd have conclusively proven it by now.

I'm going to present the case against AZT in some detail, but the essence of my opposition is quite simple: As my own physician, Dr. Joseph Sonnabend, has observed, long-term use of AZT is incompatible with life.

Every day that we live, our bodies are constantly generating new cells. DNA synthesis is the process by which new cells get formed. AZT needs to be metabolized[4] into an active compound, and in cells where this happens, AZT stops DNA synthesis wherever it finds it occurring. It doesn't differentiate between HIV-infected cells and healthy cells. In simple terms, AZT stops the body from renewing itself. For this reason, I am convinced that the use of AZT beyond twenty weeks is sheer madness.

Much of what follows is information that most AZT pushers would prefer that people with AIDS did not know. The following is not for the faint of heart. Anyone who has already decided to take AZT *no matter what* should skip to the next chapter.

MYTH 1: **All Studies of AZT Have Uniformly Drawn the Same Conclusions; There Is No Serious Disagreement About the "Benefits" of AZT.**

It is true that virtually every study of AZT has agreed on two things:

1. Many (nearly half) of people with under 200 T-helper cells can't tolerate it at all due to significant toxicity, and for those who can tolerate AZT, toxicity is probably dose-related and cumulative.[5]

2. Many (though by no means all) PWAs who can tolerate AZT experience a modest increase in T-helper cells, weight gain, and other symptom relief that generally disappears beyond twenty weeks of therapy. Frequently, T-helper cell counts return to pretreatment levels, or dip below—leaving a person worse off than when he or she began.[6]

It is *not* true that all studies support the contention that AZT extends life.

Saying that AZT can cause increases in T-helper cells that last sixteen to twenty weeks is not the same thing as saying that in the long run AZT extends life. Proponents of AZT often manipulate the confusion about the differences between short-term effects and long-term efficacy.

Explaining why he voted against approval of AZT, the chair of the FDA advisory panel that approved it explained:

There was no great difference after a while between the treated and the untreated group.[7]

PWAs who take AZT generally pay a high price in toxicity for the few weeks of increased T-cells. If these improvements were sustained over time, one might argue that the price paid is worth it. But since after sixteen to twenty weeks the T-helper cells usually decline—often dipping to *below* pretreatment levels—and since one continues to pay the price in toxicity long after any benefit has disappeared, the use of AZT beyond twenty weeks simply makes no sense.

A 1988 study[8] by Burroughs Wellcome is often cited in support of the contention that AZT extends life. However, like most studies on AZT, it is worthless. As journalist John Lauritsen has pointed out, through sheer incompetence, the Burroughs Wellcome researchers lost track of 1,120 patients—nearly a quarter of the 4,805 PWAs who received AZT. It is not possible to support the claim that AZT extends life when you don't know whether nearly a quarter of the people in your sample are dead or alive.[9]

Studies that purport to show that AZT "extends life" do outnumber those that have concluded the opposite, but evidence can be marshaled for either view. The fact that a majority of researchers believes that AZT extends life doesn't mean that it does; the issue cannot be settled by voting.

There have been two major published studies of AZT: (1) the original, American multicenter AZT trial led by Dr. Margaret Fischl[10]—the hopelessly flawed study that was the basis upon which AZT was unleashed upon the world; and (2) a slightly more extensive French study led by Dr. E. Dournon.[11] The American and French studies are of potentially equivalent value because they enrolled similarly large numbers of subjects. However, the French study is ultimately more valuable than the American study because it observed subjects over a much longer period; the American study was prematurely terminated at twenty weeks, precisely the point at which transitory improvements disappear and toxicity begins to assert itself.

Regarding the important question of design and execution, the French trial is once again superior.

The [American] study was intended to be a "double-blind placebo-controlled study," the only kind of study that can effectively prove whether or not a drug works. . . . In the case of AZT, the study became unblinded on all sides, after just a few weeks. Both sides contributed to the unblinding. It became obvious to doctors who was getting what because AZT causes such severe side effects that AIDS *per se* does not. Furthermore, a routine blood count known as a MCV [mean corpuscular volume, which is a measure of the volume of the red blood cells], which clearly shows who is on drug and who is not, wasn't whited out in the reports. Both of these facts were accepted and confirmed by both the FDA and Burroughs Wellcome, who conducted the study. Many of the patients who were in the trial admitted that they had analyzed their capsules to find out whether they were getting the drug. If they weren't, some bought the drug on the underground market. Also, the pills were supposed to be indistinguishable by taste, but they were not. . . . There were also reports that patients were pooling pills out of solidarity with each other. The study was so severely flawed that the conclusions must be considered, by the most basic scientific standards, unproven."[12]

Despite the fact that virtually everyone now acknowledges that this study was seriously flawed,[13] many still pretend that it can be used in support of AZT. A review of documents obtained under the Freedom of Information Act showed that the FDA and government researchers were well aware that there were serious flaws in the execution of the American study. However, the panel reluctantly approved AZT because of the fact that in the first sixteen weeks, nineteen people died in the placebo group while only one died in the AZT group.

This difference seems overwhelming unless one understands that the unblinding and its impact upon patient management may account for the disparate results. The reason that clinical trials are supposed to be *double*-blind is because it is recognized that a doctor may treat people receiving an experimental drug better than those who are getting placebo out of an unconscious desire to prove that the drug works. To maintain physician blinding during the AZT trial, the telltale laboratory value that indicated to physicians who was getting drug and who wasn't should have been concealed from the researchers. The fact that this was not done makes it likely that bias influenced the way patients were cared for. Since the way a PWA is cared for is probably the single greatest determinant of life and death over the short term, the seemingly dramatic survival difference between those getting AZT and those on placebo might well have been the result of bias influencing patient management.

In fact, the likelihood is great that differences in patient management accounted for the differences in the progression of the disease between the

AZT group and the placebo group. For example, in the days before PCP prophylaxis was common, whether or not a PWA died of PCP (eight out of the nineteen deaths during the trial were from PCP)[14] was a function of how quickly a diagnosis was made and how rapidly appropriate treatment was commenced. Because the errors in methodology were so egregious, it is inappropriate to attribute the difference in survival to AZT.

What is so horrifying is that the same inept researchers who were allowed to get away with such a poorly conducted trial have been permitted to repeat their mistakes. Federal trials 016 and 019, which reportedly show that AZT slows the progression of AIDS in people with ARC and who are HIV asymptomatic, suffered from the same methodological defects; according to reports, once again, the MCVs were not concealed from researchers, thus unblinding the trial.

If you don't admit your mistakes, you'll never learn from them. AIDS research is being conducted by amateurs; we deserve better than this.

Perhaps concerned that history would judge them harshly for their role in unleashing a murderous drug upon the world, the American scientists hedged their bets; they cautioned that "the initial beneficial immunologic effects of AZT may not be sustained."[15] The French study confirmed the American scientists' suspicions; it concluded that the use of AZT beyond sixteen weeks is not justified.

Referring to their results as "disappointing," the French wrote:

> The benefits of AZT are limited to a few months for ARC and AIDS patients. . . . The rationale for adhering to high-dose regimens of AZT, which in many instances leads to toxicity and interruption of treatment, seems questionable.[16]

The deafening silence in the mainstream media that followed the publication in the *Lancet* of the devastating French findings is a scandal. Despite the fact that the French study directly challenges the wisdom of using AZT as it is being widely used in the U.S., not a single major American newspaper gave prominent play to the French conclusion. Consequently, most physicians and people with AIDS remain unaware of the French study and its conclusions.

MYTH 2: **AZT Stops All HIV Replication in the Body.**

Many people are willing to endure AZT's tremendous side effects because they believe HIV activity must be stopped no matter what the cost in toxicity. In fact, many people with AIDS cope with the side effects by imagining that at least the virus is suffering as much as they are. It therefore comes as a shock to them to learn that AZT often does not reduce the amount of HIV present in the bloodstream.

The p24 antigen and antibody tests are thought by some researchers to indicate the level of active HIV replication. But at a recent conference on surrogate markers held in Washington, D.C., researchers questioned the significance of p24 data. Although there have been reports that p24 antigen declines in those on AZT, this decline occurs despite no change in the amount of free virus in the blood or in the ability to culture HIV from latently infected lymphocytes.

The question of AZT's effects on reactivation of latently infected cells is different from the question of its ability to prevent the infection of new cells. Not even the developers of AZT claim that it prevents reactivation of virus produced by latently infected cells; they claim only that AZT prevents new infections. The original American study admitted that AZT produced a "lack of measurable effect on virus isolation from peripheral-blood lymphocytes" and noted the "ability to culture virus from . . . patients after several months of [AZT] therapy."[17]

More damning is the following:

> [Only] 17 of 33 AZT recipients tested had negative [HIV] cultures at week 20. . . . There were too few subjects at week 24 of the study to allow statistically valid conclusions about an antiviral effect.[18]

The French study calls into question the widely held belief that decreases in p24 antigen levels indicate that HIV is less active *in vivo:*[19]

> Generally, in our series, full-dose AZT for two months did *not* eliminate antigenemia [HIV replication] in patients with pretreatment p24 levels of 200 units/ml or higher. Other studies have shown that after a transient fall, the level of p24 antigen can *increase* in the serum of patients with a full dose of AZT for several months.[20]

The French study is not the only one to reach this conclusion.[21]

Before deciding to subject themselves to AZT, people need to be aware that there is serious, legitimate disagreement about whether AZT reduces the amount of HIV in the bloodstream. Even Burroughs Wellcome's scientists are at a loss to explain what AZT does. "We don't know why T-4 cells go up at first, and then go down. That is one of the drug mechanisms that we are trying to understand,"[22] admitted company scientist Dr. Sandra Lehrman.

But Burroughs Wellcome scientists must not be trying very hard to understand how AZT is supposed to be working, because at a hearing held by the FDA two years after the approval of AZT, Burroughs Wellcome presented no data to support its original contention that AZT worked by interfering with HIV replication. "The claim of AZT is made on the fact that it is supposed to have an anti[retro]viral effect, and on this we have seen no data at all," said Dr. Michael Lange, one of the participants in the FDA advisory process. "Since there is a report in the *Lancet* that after 20 weeks or so, in many patients, p24 came back, do you have any data on that?"[23] he asked of the Burroughs Wellcome representative.

The Burroughs Wellcome spokesperson ducked the question by saying "What counts is the bottom line. . . . Whether you call it better because of some antiviral effect, or some other antibacterial effect, they [the patients on AZT] are still better."[24]

MYTH 3: AZT increases T-Helper Cells.

There is no disagreement that AZT frequently produces modest increases in T-helper cells during the first sixteen to twenty weeks of therapy in those who can tolerate it at all. But there is also no disagreement that for most people with AIDS who continue to take full-dose AZT beyond twenty weeks, these transitory improvements disappear.

Instead of increasing T-helper cells, AZT probably *kills* T-helper cells. The French study observed that

> in some studies, including ours, the decrease of [T-helper] cell counts below the initial value after a few months of AZT suggests that this drug might be toxic to [T-helper] cells.[25]

Since AZT is a DNA-chain terminator, it kills many cells—not just T-helper cells. Professor Peter Duesberg states the case against AZT bluntly. As a chemotherapeutic agent, AZT "kills dividing blood cells and other cells [and is thus] directly immunosuppressive."[26]

In principle AZT is a bad drug, if for no other reason than it impairs one of the most important needs of someone with AIDS: the capacity to regenerate new T-helper cells.

MYTH 4: AZT Prolongs Life by Reducing the Incidence and Severity of Opportunistic Infections.

At a forum held in November 1988 at Columbia University, New York researcher Dr. Craig Metroka presented an overview of the use of AZT in AIDS. The evidence he gave directly contradicts the oft-repeated contention that AZT extends life by preventing opportunistic infections. Evidence presented by other forum participants corroborated Dr. Metroka's assertion.

For example, one researcher presented findings from a Memorial Sloan-Kettering study that had lasted a year and a half and that had followed 247 people with full-blown AIDS, 74 percent of whom used AZT for an average of 7.8 months:

> By 15 months, 80 percent of people on AZT *not receiving [PCP] prophylaxis* had a recurrent episode of pneumocystis. Among patients receiving aerosol pentamidine, only 5 percent in the 15-month period . . . developed a recurring episode [of PCP]. This is a 16-fold reduction."[27]

So, AZT doesn't do much to prevent PCP. In fact, there is some evidence to suggest that AZT *increases* one's likelihood of developing PCP:

> Initial reports of the benefits of [AZT] therapy for HIV infection indicated a decreased incidence of [opportunistic infections]. Optimistic authors hypothesized that zidovudine alone might obviate the need for prophylaxis of AIDS-related OIs. Unfortunately, the incidence of recurrent PCP remains little changed by zidovudine therapy without secondary prophylaxis. In an ongoing prospective study, recurrent PCP has been diagnosed in 272 of 561 (48.5 percent) nonprophylaxed patients receiving [AZT] over a 10-month mean follow-up period. Similarly, in a retrospective analysis, *the mean time to PCP recurrence was noted to be 28.5 weeks among 16 patients receiving [AZT] compared to 35.8 weeks among 55 patients not receiving [AZT].*[28]

In other words, people who were not on any form of PCP prevention therapy but who were taking AZT developed another bout of PCP seven weeks *sooner* than did nonprophylaxed PWAs who weren't taking AZT. A recently published article[29] by Dr. A. Bruce Montgomery strongly suggests that AZT *increases* one's risk for a second bout of PCP in those not receiving any form of PCP prophylaxis. A whopping 32 percent of 318 nonprophylaxing AZT users developed a second bout of PCP by six months, as compared with only 18 percent of 201 PWAs receiving neither AZT nor PCP prophylaxis. By one year after the first bout of PCP, the percentages of recurrence for each group were 68 percent versus 46 percent, respectively.

Such findings strongly support two observations. First, the increases in survival time for PWAs that most people are attributing to the introduction of AZT are more probably due to PCP prophylaxis. PCP prophylaxis became widely practiced in 1987—the same time that AZT was introduced. Second, because of its clearly established ability to kill precisely those T-helper cells that PWAs so desperately need more of, this evidence strongly suggests that AZT is exacerbating the underlying immunosuppression instead of correcting it.

What about KS? Forum participant Dr. Metroka was blunt and succinct: "AZT probably has no direct effect on the rate of development of Kaposi's sarcoma."[30]

What about lymphoma? AZT was invented as cancer chemotherapy in the sixties, but was abandoned as a failure. Not only is there no evidence that AZT prevents lymphoma and other cancers, but there is evidence that AZT *causes* cancer. In fact, government researchers have reported that of the nineteen patients in the original Phase I AZT trial, three developed lymphoma within two and a half years, an incidence far in excess of what one would expect in AIDS.[31]

AZT "should not be used as a sole treatment for a lymphoma," cautioned Dr. Metroka. He further warned against using AZT for patients also receiving cancer chemotherapy:

> Even half-doses of AZT can lead to the development of life-threatening drops in white blood cell count [when used in conjunction with other] chemotherapeutic agents which have minimal bone marrow toxicity.

So, with the possible exception of a beneficial effect upon neurological complications of AIDS, AZT does not have a significant impact on the incidence of the major opportunistic complications. AZT doesn't prevent—and shouldn't be used to treat—the most common opportunistic complications of AIDS.

MYTH 5: The Benefits of Long-Term Use of AZT Outweigh the Risks.

San Francisco's Project Inform is the most prominent AIDS activist organization pushing AZT. Through public speaking engagements and the worldwide distribution of its information packets, PI has encouraged thousands of people to take AZT.

Its fact sheet on AZT contains the following:

> It has become popular to argue against the value of AZT because of the seriousness of its side effects, because it is not a cure, and because it is so incredibly overpriced. However, these factors must be placed in perspective. In the overall picture, AZT is helping great numbers of people, at least for a time. It is readily apparent that the quality of life for most AIDS patients is much better than it was 2 years ago. Some of the credit must go to AZT. We do ourselves a disservice if we overstate its drawbacks while undervaluing its benefits. Many patients couldn't be happier with the drug. Based on all the evidence, it offers seriously ill people greater likelihood of help than any other alternative. We say this as one of AZT's first, loudest, and best-informed critics. The challenge is learning how and when to use it, and how and when to stop using it.[32]

How is it possible to overstate the drawbacks of AZT? What is being overstated are its benefits! The truth is, we know a great deal more about the risks of AZT than we do about the supposed benefits.

There is simply no question that AZT is an incredibly toxic drug. AZT was invented as a potential cancer agent. According to its inventor, Jerome Horwitz, "[AZT is] cytotoxic, and as such, it causes bone marrow toxicity and anemia." With breathtaking understatement, he admitted: "There are problems with the drug. It's not perfect."[33]

Most chemotherapy is toxic and immunosuppressive. The difference between AZT and most cancer chemotherapeutic agents is that chemotherapy is intended to be used in short, intense bursts designed to kill the cancer before it kills the patient. The idea that individuals should take chemotherapy every day for the rest of their lives is completely unprecedented.

"I can't see how this drug could be doing anything other than making people very sick,"[34] said Dr. Harvey Bialy, scientific editor of the journal *Biotechnology*.

Professor Peter Duesberg, a member of the prestigious National Academy of Sciences and one of the world's foremost experts on retroviruses, concurs: "[AZT] ends up killing millions of lymphocytes. It's beyond me how that could possibly be beneficial."[35]

Cancer is, in a sense, the exact opposite of AIDS. Cancer is characterized by the uncontrollable *over* production of cells. AIDS is defined as the *depletion* of key cells of the immune system. What sense does it make to treat a disease defined by the loss of T-cells with a drug designed to kill them, and which also prevents new cells from forming?

Bone marrow is the source of new T-cells, and even the most ardent AZT booster acknowledges that a major side effect of AZT is bone-marrow suppression.

Those who are convinced that AZT extends life for several months or more might argue that giving AZT to someone with full-blown AIDS is justified. If we assume for the sake of argument that AZT enables a desperately ill PWA to live twenty weeks longer than he or she otherwise would have, it might be reasonable to conclude that the risks of potential long-term toxicity, including cancer, are outweighed by this benefit. One might persuasively argue that for people who have a life expectancy of not more than two years, the potential risks of bone-marrow suppression and cancer may be offset by the potential benefit of extending life a few months.

But the risk/benefit analysis is very different when one considers prescribing AZT to healthy, asymptomatic HIV seropositives with the intent that they take the drug for the rest of their lives. AZT is now being prescribed for people who are asymptomatic and who presumably have many years to live. The risk that the long-term use of AZT might kill T-helper cells and cause cancer is very real and must be factored into the risk/benefit equation.[36]

Dr. Brook, chair of the FDA panel and the only member to vote *against* the approval of AZT, warned:

> The side effects were so very severe. It was chemotherapy. Patients were going to need blood transfusions. That's very serious. [Approving it prematurely would be like] letting the genie out of the bottle.[37]

The genie is now very much out of the bottle. The panel's fear that AZT might be prescribed for essentially healthy people has come true.

One doubts that even the FDA reviewers who approved AZT could have imagined that this drug would one day be given to pregnant women and to HIV-antibody-positive infants!

Another risk associated with AZT that has been ignored or downplayed is the possibility that it causes cancer. Even Dr. Samuel Broder, the government scientist who claims the dubious credit for unleashing AZT upon the world, has acknowledged the distinct possibility that AZT causes cancer:

> In considering early intervention with [AZT], it is of particular concern that the drug may be carcinogenic or mutagenic; its long-term effects are unknown. . . . Lymphomas developed in 3 of our original 19 Phase I patients between 1 and 2½ years after Zidovudine therapy began (unpublished data).[38]

In his incisive expose entitled "AZT and Cancer," journalist John Lauritsen presented the findings of FDA toxicologist Harvey I. Chernov, Ph.D., who recommended *against* the approval of AZT on the basis of toxicity:

> Dose-related chromosome damage was observed in an *in vitro* cytogenetic assay using human lymphocytes. . . . This behavior is characteristic of tumor cells and suggests that AZT may be a potential carcinogen. It appears to be at least as active as the . . . control material, methylcholanthrene [a known and extremely potent carcinogen].[39]

Burroughs Wellcome attempted to downplay the probability that AZT causes cancer by proposing that the labeling insert should obfuscate as follows: "The significance of these *in vitro* results is not known." To his tremendous credit, Chernov strenuously objected to Burroughs Wellcome's patently disingenuous attempt to obscure the drug's potential carcinogenicity:

> The sentence: "The significance of these *in vitro* results is not known" is not accurate. A test chemical which induces a positive response in the cell transformation assay is presumed to be a potential carcinogen.[40]

Unfortunately, Burroughs Wellcome successfully counterproposed labeling language that is just as obscure and misleading as its original proposal. Very few people who are taking AZT are ever told that it might cause cancer and that its potential to cause cancer probably increases with dose and duration.

According to Dr. Ellen Cooper of the FDA, the unprecedented rapid approval of AZT represented a "significant and potentially dangerous departure from our normal toxicology requirements."[41]

I predict that the approval of AZT will prove to be a scandal of the magnitude of thalidomide. Years from now, when AIDS has been cured, I predict that people who took AZT are going to turn up with high rates of cancer. No doubt another epidemic will be declared and the cancer will be attributed to anything but its true cause: AZT. Subsequent events suggest Dr. Cooper's concerns were justified.

The FDA is supposed to make certain that no drug gets released in America until it has been proven both safe and effective. But with AIDS, standard caution gets cast aside.[42] At the same time the FDA was warning Americans about the dangers of Red Dye No. 5, it cooperated in a mind-boggling attempt to downplay the ominous results of a study of AZT carcigenicity in rodents. In what appeared to be an attempt to limit future liability without risking the projected multibillion-dollar market for AZT,[43] Burroughs Wellcome sent a mailing to every physician in the United States notifying them that the results of "routine tests carried out on new drugs" found that "there was an incidence of vaginal squamous cell carcinoma formation toward the end of the life span of rodents treated with high doses of zidovudine."[44]

In a shocking display of how easy it is to find an AIDS expert who will say anything, a bevy of so-called AIDS experts took to the press to support the contention of Burroughs Wellcome that "the clinical significance of these findings or the need to alter current zidovudine therapy is not apparent as tumorigenicity in rodents is not necessarily associated with carcinogenicity in humans."[45]

If "tumorigenicity in rodents is not necessarily associated with carcinogenicity in humans," why does the FDA require such studies to be done and why did Burroughs Wellcome feel compelled to send out a "Dear Doctor" letter? At a minimum, women who are taking AZT should seriously consider the gender-specific carcigenicity of AZT when given to rodents.

Finally, there is at least one other major side effect that most people taking AZT are not aware of: impotence. I first became aware of the fact that AZT may cause impotence after giving a speech in Seattle, Washington. A person with AIDS who had been taking full-dose AZT for a year burst into a PWA support group that I was attending while on a trip to Seattle. He was extremely agitated, having just come from his doctor's office.

He proceeded to tell a frightening story. About a year after starting

AZT, for the first time in his life, he was unable to have an erection. He immediately went to his doctor to ask if his impotence might be AZT-related. He insisted that his doctor call Burroughs Wellcome.

According to him, as he secretly listened on an extension, his doctor asked the scientists at Burroughs Wellcome whether they had ever heard of AZT causing impotence. They reportedly said that yes, it was a quite common side effect. Startled, the doctor asked why impotence wasn't listed as a side effect in the *Physicians' Desk Reference*. The Burroughs Wellcome representatives hemmed and hawed. The doctor began to get angry and said, "Don't you think that people with AIDS should be told they might become impotent if they take AZT?" According to the PWA, they responded in essence, "These people shouldn't be having sex anyway." The PWA was furious and announced his intention to file a class-action lawsuit on behalf of all PWAs who have experienced impotence as the result of AZT.

I was surprised that someone as opposed to AZT as me hadn't heard that impotence was a common side effect. So I decided to check it out. I asked how many other men in the Seattle support group were on full-dose AZT. About sixteen people raised their hands. I asked how many of them had been on full dose for at least a year. Twelve kept their hands raised. I asked how many of those dozen were impotent. The number shocked me: all twelve.

All hell broke loose. People started talking all at once and the anger began to mount. They floated the idea of holding an AZT speak-out to alert other PWAs to the problem of drug-induced impotence.

Several said they had assumed their impotence was the result of AIDS, not AZT. When I thought about it, it made sense that I had never heard that impotence might be a side effect of AZT. Most people don't talk about impotence; it's embarrassing. And others might have imagined—or been told by their doctors—that their impotence was the result of AIDS.

If the other reasons not to take AZT aren't sufficient, perhaps the prospect of impotence will make people think twice about giving in to the AZT frenzy.

⊠ FINAL THOUGHTS

There is another unrecognized side effect of AZT that also needs to be considered. The so-called "success" of AZT has made it very difficult to test other drugs. It is considered unethical to ask someone to try an experimental drug or risk getting a placebo, since AZT has been "proven" to prevent the progression of AIDS. Therefore all federal studies that were in the planning stages when AZT was approved had to be redesigned to include AZT.

According to ACT-UP analysis of federal AIDS drug trials, over 90 percent of the subjects in current government AIDS trials are taking AZT and similar antiretroviral drugs. This has led to discrimination against those of us who have decided not to take AZT or who cannot tolerate it. To enter a clinical trial of another drug, we either have to prove that we are AZT-intolerant or risk getting AZT as a placebo.

Another unfortunate side effect of AZT is that it has been used to obscure the abject failure of the federal research effort. Federal bureaucrats point to the rapid approval of AZT as an example of how the system can work and as proof that they are responsive and compassionate. As long as activists could shout that the federal government hadn't produced a single treatment for the treatment of AIDS, it was easy to make the case for increased government spending on AIDS research. But now that most AIDS activists have uncritically accepted government claims that AZT extends life, there is less urgency to find drugs that really work. If AIDS has already become the chronic, manageable disease that some activists and government officials are now claiming it is, we are likely to witness increasingly strident claims that too much money is being spent on AIDS in relation to other diseases.

AZT was foisted upon us based on the claim that it worked in a straightforward way: It was supposed to stop HIV replication. It is amazing to me that Burroughs Wellcome and government researchers now admit AZT may not affect the amount of HIV present in the blood. In fact, they haven't got any plausible explanation of how AZT is supposed to be working.

Undoubtedly AZT is having some effect on people with AIDS; something must be responsible for the transitory improvements. If AZT's mechanism of action is not in fact anti-retroviral, might not the "benefits" of AZT, such as they are, be attributable to other effects that might be achievable with drugs of significantly less toxicity? Why aren't we trying to find out?

AIDS expert Dr. Michael Lange has suggested that AZT's benefits may be attributable to an antiinflammatory effect. Drugs such a indomethacin, a nonsteroidal antiinfalmmatory, can achieve this with significantly less toxicity. Aspirin is another antiinflammatory that might produce similar results.

My doctor suggests that the temporary improvements attributable to AZT may even be the result of the frequent transfusions made necessary by AZT anemia. (A researcher at St. Luke's Hospital in New York has proposed that transfusions help the body remove immune complexes.) Dr. Sonnabend also points out that

> AZT might exert an effect by a direct antimicrobial action on opportunistic pathogens. . . . AZT does inhibit Epstein-Barr virus (EBV). . . . AZT is also highly active against a group of gram negative bacteria, including salmonella and shigella, although there is no reason to believe that this activity [is] of clinical benefit.[46]

There are definitely less toxic ways than AZT to remove immune complexes, inhibit EBV, and destroy salmonella and shigella. For example, acyclovir—a relatively nontoxic drug used to prevent herpes reactivations—deserves to be studied as a treatment for AIDS, since it is generally recognized that herpes virus reactivations play a major role in the progression of AIDS. Sadly, there are apparently no AIDS-related trials of acyclovir that do not combine it with AZT.

The case against AZT would not be complete without some mention of its obscene price. Without including the costs of the blood work necessary to monitor for signs of toxicity, or the cost of transfusions it often makes necessary, AZT is one of the most expensive drugs in the world. And it was developed largely at taxpayer expense.

The outrageous price would be bad enough if the drug actually worked; but given the conflicting evidence, the money spent on AZT squanders a resource that might better be applied to finding a real cure for AIDS. It has been tremendously frustrating for those of us who oppose the use of AZT to see fellow AIDS activists support the transfer of $5 million from AIDS research funding to make AZT available to those who can't afford it.

Finally, some have suggested that AZT is a good drug that has been poorly used.

In February 1990, the recommended dose of AZT was reduced by half. While this is definitely good news, since AZT's fabled toxicity appears to be dose-related, a number of questions are raised by this dose reduction.

First, what took so long? People with AIDS, and community physicians taking care of them, learned the hard way—through trial and error—that the original dose was way too high.

Second, how was the original dose chosen? Why was it so high? Common sense ought to have dictated that with a drug known to be as toxic as AZT, the goal should have been to find the lowest possible "effective" dose. How must those PWAs feel who suffered the horrific side effects and endless transfusions necessitated by full-dose AZT?

Third, there are rumors among AIDS activists that government researchers have yet to find a dose of AZT so low that "efficacy" is lost. In other words, if 500 milligrams is as "efficacious" as 1,000, might not 250 or 125 or 50 milligrams a day be just as "effective"? Given the profit that Burroughs Wellcome is making, how likely is it that these questions are being asked? And if they're being asked, how reasonable is it to expect that we'll have an answer any time soon?

If I was convinced that taking AZT was my best chance of surviving AIDS, I'd do my own clinical trial on myself. I'd start with 50 milligrams a day and watch my numbers. Since I suspect that many of the benefits being attributable to AZT are really placebo effects, it would be interesting to see how many PWAs respond well to 50 milligrams a day. With AZT, less, as they say, is very definitely more.

In any event, PWAs who are taking AZT should keep themselves up-to-date on the latest scuttlebutt about lowering the dosage of AZT yet further. My prediction is that rather than admit that AZT has been a fraud from start to finish, we will witness the gradual reduction of the dose until one day, quietly and without fanfare, it reaches zero.

⊠ If I saw a friend about to drink a glass of Drano, I would without hesitation knock it from his hand. I consider AZT to be Drano in pill form—pure, lethal poison. Anyone who takes AZT without examining *all* the evidence is a fool.

I know my comparison of AZT and Drano outrages many people, and I do not mean to be glib. But I have searched in vain for some other way to effectively express the depth of my conviction that we are headed down a very dangerous road. I have seen the devastation wreaked by AZT. I have also watched in horror as PWAs turn the color of boiled ham from AZT poisoning, endure the melting away of their muscles, become transfusion-dependent, and experience drug-induced psychosis. And all this suffering is caused by a drug that was abandoned as unfit for human use more than a decade ago.

The claim that only crazy people—or individuals with some suspect agenda—question the wisdom of AZT use is evidence of the inability of those promoting its use to answer calmly and rationally the case against it. Deciding whether to take this powerfully toxic drug may well determine whether you live or die. Don't allow yourself to be influenced by strident, desperate bullies who believe that you aren't capable of making the right decision on the basis of all available data.

Questioning the value of AZT evokes ferocious denunciations and hostility. Much of the fury directed at critics of AZT is actually displaced frustration over the fact that entering the second decade of AIDS, people are forced to make life-and-death treatment choices on the basis of data that is soft, contradictory, and inconclusive.

Desperate for some certainty, most people are reluctant to admit that the evidence in support of the contention that AZT extends life is about as reliable as the evidence that, say, lipids extend life. There's certainly *more* data about AZT, but in the final analysis, the evidence is about as soft as that for other therapies. Contrary to the Project Inform party line, we do ourselves a disservice if we overstate AZT's benefits while undervaluing its drawbacks.

If the data ever changes and a *convincing* case can be made that the benefits of AZT outweigh its harms, I'll admit I was wrong and be first in line to get my prescription filled. Till that unlikely day, I intend to persist in presenting the strong case against zidovudine. Because as far as I can see, few, if any, can survive both AIDS and AZT.

NOTES

1. Unfortunately, we have no way of knowing whether or not the fact that they haven't taken AZT may be *responsible* for their being alive. If they are like the long-term survivors I've interviewed, the odds are that they aren't on AZT; that may be an important part of why they continue to survive and thrive more than a decade after diagnosis.

2. Farber, Celia, "Sins of Omission: The AZT Scandal," *Spin*, 5, no. 8 (November 1989): 115.

3. Cotton, Paul, "Controversy Continues as Experts Ponder Zidovudine's Role in Early HIV Infection." *JAMA*, 263, no. 12 (March 23, 1990): 1605.

4. It is theoretically quite plausible that the few individuals who have been able to tolerate AZT without significant side effects may in fact be deficient in their ability to metabolize AZT. This may be a blessing in disguise, although it would no doubt pain such an individual to think that $10,000 worth of medication is simply being flushed through the system.

5. Because the mean and median time on AZT was a mere 120 and 127 days (19 to 20 weeks), respectively, the American study appropriately cautioned that, "[s]ince the present observations were made over only 24 weeks, the long-term benefits and toxic effects of AZT in this patient population still need to be defined."

The French study found that more than half of all people on AZT had to discontinue taking it or had to reduce the dose due to significant toxicity.

6. The American study cited in Farber's *Spin* article found that

[a]fter 12 weeks of therapy, a gradual decline in the number of [T-helper] cells was noted in those with AIDS who were receiving AZT and who remained in the study; after 20 weeks, a return to base-line values occurred in many of these subjects. . . .

The absolute number of CD4 cells decreased after 20 weeks in many subjects with a diagnosis of AIDS . . . suggesting that the initial beneficial immunologic effects of AZT may not be sustained.

The French study likewise confirmed that for most people, the improvements disappear after about 20 weeks:

By six months, these [improved laboratory] values had returned to their pretreatment levels and several opportunisitic infections, malignancies and deaths occurred. ["Effects of Zidovudine in 365 Consecutive Patients with AIDS or AIDS-Related Complex," see note 16 below.]

If the American study had not been terminated prematurely, it would have reached the same conclusions as the French study. According to Dr. Itzhak Brook, the chair of the FDA advisory panel that approved AZT and the only member to vote *against* approval, the death rate in the group receiving AZT accelerated shortly after the study was stopped:

There was no great difference after a while between the treated and the untreated group. [Dr. Itzhak Brook, quoted in "Sins of Omission."]

7. Farber, "Sins of Omission," 44.

8. Creagh-Kirk, Terri, et al., "Survival Experience Among Patients with AIDS Receiving Zidovudine: Follow-up of Patients in a Compassionate Plea Program," *JAMA* (November 25, 1988).

9. For a fuller critique of this study, see John Lauritsen's appropriately scathing deconstruction "On the AZT Front: Part Two," *New York Native* (January 16, 1989): 16–19.

10. Fischl, Margaret A., "The Efficacy of Azidothymidine (AZT) in the Treatment of Patients with AIDS and AIDS-Related Complex: A Double-Blind, Placebo-Controlled Trial," *New England Journal of Medicine,* 317 (July 23, 1987): 185–91.

11. Dournon, E., et al., "Effects of Zidovudine in 365 Consecutive Patients with AIDS or AIDS-Related Complex," *Lancet,* 2 (December 3, 1988): 1297.

12. Farber, "Sins of Omission," 42.

13. For a devastating critique of the American AZT trial, read "Review of AZT Multicenter Trial Data Obtained Under the Freedom of Information Act by Project Inform and ACT-UP," written and privately circulated in October 1987 by Dr. Joseph A. Sonnabend, and subsequently published in *AIDS Forum,* 1 (January 1989).

14. The purpose of doing a multicenter trial is to see if you get the same results in each center. If not, it suggests that there may have been differences in execution. In fact, none of the nineteen deaths that occurred in the placebo arm occurred in New York. This suggests that people with AIDS in New York were being looked after by

community physicians who wouldn't allow their patients to die from PCP within sixteen weeks following a previous episode of PCP.

15. Fischl, op. cit.

16. Dournon, 1301–1302.

17. Fischl, op. cit.

18. Fischl, op. cit.

19. At an NIH-sponsored conference on surrogate markers held in Washington in the fall of 1989, it was generally agreed that p24 was not a useful measure of anything. Many, perhaps most, people with AIDS don't have p24, and for those that did, reductions in p24 did not correlate with actual HIV replication. Despite the consensus reached at this conference that p24 is not a useful marker of a drug's efficacy, many segments of the AIDS activist community continue to clamor for wider access to p24 testing.

20. Dournon, op. cit. (emphasis added).

21. See Gupta, P., et al., "Cell-to-Cell Transmission of Human Immunodeficiency Virus Type I in the Presence of Azidothymidine and Neutralizing Antibody," *Journal of Virology,* 63 (May 1989): 2361, which states, "AZT and virus-neutralizing antibody had no effect on cell-to-cell transmission of HIV-1."

22. Farber, "Sins of Omission," 44.

23. Farber, ibid.

24. Farber, "Sins of Omission," 115.

25. Dournon, op. cit.

26. Farber, "Sins of Omission," 44.

27. Transcript, Columbia Gay Health Advocacy Project, "AIDS: Improving the Odds 1988," New York, 1989.

28. Hardy, W. David, M.D., "Prophylaxis of AIDS-Related Opportunistic Infections (OIs)," in *The 1989 AIDS Clinical Review,* edited by Paul Volberding, M.D., and Mark Jacobson, M.D. (New York: Marcel Dekker, 1989), 125–50. Emphasis added.

29. Montgomery, A. Bruce, M.D., "Prophylaxis of *Pneumocystic Carinii* Pneumonia in Patients Infected with the Human Immunodeficiency Virus Type 1," *Seminars in Respiratory Infections,* 4, 4 (December 1989): 311–317.

30. "AIDS: Improving the Odds 1988," see note 27.

31. Varchoan, Robert, Mitsuya, Hiroaki, Myers, Charles E., and Broder, Samuel, "Clinical Pharmacology of 3'-Azido-2'3'-Dideoxythymidine (Zidovudine) and Related Dideoxynucleosides," *New England Journal of Medicine* (September 14, 1989): 726–735.

32. From "Project Inform Fact Sheet on AZT," reprinted in *Positive Living,* published by The People Living With AIDS program (VIC) of the Victorian AIDS Council/Gay Men's Health Center (Collingwood, Australia), 1989.

33. Farber, ibid.

34. Farber, ibid.

35. Farber, ibid.

36. As I write this in April 1990, the federal government is aggressively encouraging healthy, asymptomatic HIV-seropositive individuals with T-helper cell counts as high as 500 to take 500 milligrams of AZT a day for the rest of their lives. The results of several trials claiming to demonstrate that this dose of AZT slows the progression of AIDS were announced at a press conference. I'm pleased to report that a number of physicians have expressed their disgust at being asked to write prescriptions by press release.

U.S. government officials remain undaunted by the increasingly frequent criticisms of AZT. A recent article by Laurie Garrett of *New York Newsday* [Garrett, Laura, "Many Not Using AIDS Drug AZT," *New York Newsday* (April 5, 1990):15] quotes top AIDS researcher Dr. Anthony Fauci lamenting the fact that healthy HIV-seropositives were not rushing like lemmings to the sea to poison themselves with AZT.

Garrett writes:

According to the research findings, about 40 percent of all people infected with HIV, the AIDS virus, should consider taking AZT. That translates into about 650,000 nationwide and an estimated 40,000 to 140,000 New Yorkers. National AZT-use figures are not readily available, but New York state officials said yesterday only 13,000 mostly low-income people receive free AZT through state and federally funded programs, including Medicaid, and an unknown smaller number obtain the drug through private insurance. . . . Nationwide, authorities estimate that if all asymptomatic HIV-infected individuals who would qualify for AZT under the current program were to obtain it, drug expenditure would exceed $1 billion.

Garrett's article quotes several researchers and government representatives speculating as to why more people aren't taking AZT. The only explanation anyone can seem to think of is a "reluct[ance] to know the [HIV antibody] test results and fears [about] the stigmas attached to an HIV diagnosis." No acknowledgment is made of the fact that many individuals remain skeptical about the "benefits" of AZT.

I would argue that there are two more important reasons that might account for such apparently widespread skepticism: (1) Most people at risk for AIDS know someone who has taken AZT; they've seen firsthand that any temporary benefits experienced by those who can tolerate AZT at all are swiftly canceled out by its horrendous side effects; and (2) most people knowledgeable about the sordid history of AIDS treatment research know instinctively to distrust anything that federal researchers say.

Skepticism about the wisdom of prescribing AZT for essentially healthy HIV-seropositive persons has received enormous support from researchers in Europe. According to a recent *Journal of the American Medical Association (JAMA)* article:

Maxime Seligmann, M.D., protocol chair of the French arm of the Concorde 1 trial of [AZT] in asymptomatic patients . . . says his study's data safety monitoring board had concluded that the NIAID data do not justify closing Concorde's placebo arm.

Several letters written by European researchers harshly critical of the American studies have been published in several prestigious medical journals. It seems clear that the European AIDS research community shares the view of many that the American data that we've been told at a press conference convincingly demonstrates that AZT significantly delays the progression of AIDS is not, in fact, very compelling.

Another harsh critic of the NIAID study is John D. Hamilton, M.D., cochair of a Veterans Administration study of AZT. According to the *JAMA* article:

> [A]nalysis at 2 years demonstrated "no statistically significant difference in progression to AIDS" for patients in the 200 to 500 CD4 cell count range and that deaths in both treatment and placebo cohorts are "virtually identical."

Any HIV-seropositive individual who is facing the difficult decision about whether or not to start on AZT should make sure that she or he keeps abreast of the latest reports about the battles between American and European researchers over the "benefits" of AZT.

37. Farber, "Sins of Omission," 42.

38. Varchoan, op. cit., 731.

39. Chernov, Harvey, Ph.D., "Review and Evaluation of Pharmacology and Toxicology Data [on AZT]," submitted to the FDA on December 29, 1986, quoted in John Lauritsen, "AZT and Cancer," *New York Native* (October 30, 1988): 14. I strongly urge anyone who wishes to stay truly informed about AIDS to follow the writings of feisty reporter John Lauritsen. A collection of his AZT critiques has been published as *Poison by Prescription: The AZT Story* (New York: Asklepios, 1990).

40. Lauritsen, "AZT and Cancer," 15.

41. Dr. Ellen Cooper of the FDA, quoted in Celia Farber, "Sins of Omission."

42. A recent *New York Times* article bluntly acknowledged that scientific standards get lowered when the issue is AIDS. Referring to the recent FDA approval of AZT for use in treating children, the article stated that:

> Members of the [FDA advisory] panel . . . said that available data on the safety and effectiveness of AZT in children did not meet agency requirements. But for the first time in agency history, they voted to take advantage of an FDA rule allowing them to waive the Federal standards in cases of life-threatening children's disease. . . . Several members of the advisory committee were highly critical of the data presented by the company. One panelist . . . accused the company of 'stacking the deck' in favor of approval.

[From "FDA Panel Urges AZT for Children: Agency's Approval Is Expected—Advisors Act in Spite of Doubts on AIDS Drug," a Reuters dispatch that ran in the *New York Times* (March 31, 1990): A-10.]

I'm afraid that AIDS activists bear some responsibility for scandalous lowering of scientific standards taking place at the FDA. Those activists whose rallying cry is "Drugs into bodies" often mean "Any drug into anybody, regardless of toxicity." Some activists appear to be urging a total deregulation of the drug industry.

It is virtually universally agreed that the current FDA system of drug approval is cumbersome, inefficient, and inadequate to the task of finding safe and effective therapies for AIDS in an appropriately expeditious fashion. It does not follow, however, that the best solution is total deregulation. One can argue that the FDA could relax its standards for proving efficacy in a life-threatening disease such as AIDS; but I consider it disastrous to abandon the FDA's traditional concern for toxicity. We abandon all caution at our own peril.

43. For a discussion of the enormous profits which Burroughs Wellcome stands to make from AZT, see Freudenheim, Milt, "Big Gain Seen for Owner of AZT Maker," *New York Times* (August 19, 1989).

44. See the "Backgrounder" document titled "Zidovudine: Results of Rodent Life-time Carcinogenicity Studies," issued by Burroughs Wellcome Co. on December 5, 1989. This "Backgrounder" was included along with a "Dear Doctor" letter mailed on December 5 and signed by David W. Barry, M.D., Vice President of Research, Development and Medical, for Burroughs Wellcome Co.

45. "Backgrounder," ibid.

46. Sonnabend, "Review of AZT Multicenter Trial Data Obtained Under the Freedom of Information Act by Project Inform and ACT-UP," op. cit.

LIVING IS THE BEST REVENGE

⊠⊠⊠ Yes, attitude matters. But ultimately, controlling AIDS is going to require finding the right combination of drugs.

There are two major reasons to believe that many PWAs may live to collect retirement benefits:

1. Patient management continues to improve dramatically; in particular, major breakthroughs in the prevention of the opportunistic diseases besides PCP are imminent; and

2. The community-based research movement may soon explore a non-HIV based, multimodal treatment regimen that may be the cure we've all been waiting for.

Patient Management

Most people believe that curing AIDS will depend upon finding a magic bullet. Visions of Nobel prizes dance in the heads of government AIDS researchers. But absent a cure, the main determinant of a PWA's survival is the nonglamorous, labor-intensive patient care being quietly provided every day by heroic community physicians.

Proper patient management has two main components: (1) prophylaxis to prevent opportunistic infections in the first place; and (2) the aggressive diagnosis and treatment of infections that do occur. The ultimate goal of proper patient management is to keep patients alive until a cure is found.

Surviving AIDS requires access to an experienced, compassionate, knowledgeable physician who hasn't bought into the myth that there's no point in aggressively diagnosing and treating opportunistic complications since everyone with AIDS is doomed. The doctors who early on risked the scorn of their colleagues by insisting that their patients take medication to prevent PCP have made the most important contribution to long-term survival. It's the physicians who see to it that their patients have proper nutrition and psychosocial support and who encourage their patients to try nontoxic drugs first who deserve much of the credit for the steadily improving survival figures.

Prospects for Preventing Opportunistic Infections

The most important aspect of proper AIDS patient management is the prevention of opportunistic infections. The theory behind prophylaxis is that it's easier and preferable to prevent a disease in the first place than to try to treat it after it occurs. Community-based research into prophylaxis is currently under way; the goal is to take drugs known to be effective in treating a particular opportunistic infection and then find the lowest possible dosage which, when taken prophylactically, will be safe and effective at preventing the particular infection. As AIDS researcher Jonathan Gold, M.D., recently observed in an AIDS newsletter, "The importance, high frequency, and relative ease of study of the infectious complications of AIDS should make development of prophylactic measures a high priority."[1]

Some people with AIDS, after seeking the opinion of their physicians, aren't waiting for the results of the research; many have already begun to experiment with low doses of the drugs mentioned in the following overview. Since toxicity and drug interaction are always important concerns, PWAs should never proceed willy-nilly to take a drug or drugs without proper supervision.

Five infections—PCP, CMV, MAI, toxoplasmosis, and cryptococcal meningitis—occur in at least 80 percent of people with AIDS.[2] If in the near future community researchers can demonstrate that certain drugs at certain doses prevent these lethal diseases, tens of thousands of people with AIDS might be kept alive long enough to benefit from a cure for the underlying immune deficiency itself.

Hopefully, by the time this book is published, the Community Research

Initiative of New York (an organization on whose board of directors I serve) will have issued detailed interim guidelines for the prophylaxis of the following opportunistic infections. PWAs should make sure their physicians keep up to date on the latest recommendations for caring for people with AIDS.

What follows is an overview of the exciting research currently being planned or conducted by community-based research groups around the country. Any person with AIDS who is looking for some reason to stay alive should keep a list of promising community-based clinical trials by the bed.

Pneumocystis Carinii Pneumonia

As discussed throughout this book, the success of PCP prophylaxis, coupled with major advances in treatment of PCP infection, essentially means that no one with AIDS should die from PCP. Anyone at high risk for PCP should have her or his immune system regularly monitored and PCP prophylaxis should be initiated if the number of T-helper cells dips below 200; one can argue that any person with AIDS who dies of PCP these days was murdered by medical incompetence.

Now we have the luxury of comparing whether systemic PCP prophylaxis (with sulfa drugs such as Bactrim, Fansidar, and dapsone) is preferable to aerosol pentamidine. Unfortunately, many people are allergic to sulfa drugs, although physicians are exploring ways to reduce allergic reactions.[3] For those who can tolerate it, Bactrim offers the advantage of providing protection against other infections, such as salmonella, shigella, pneumococcus, and Haemophilus influenzae.[4]

The prophylactic use of aerosol pentamidine is also being refined. Community-based researchers are investigating "the best frequency of administration, optimal nebulizer, dose and posture and breathing method for inhaling the aerosolized mist."[5]

Cytomegalovirus (CMV)

Finding drugs that can control CMV infection is an urgent priority for two reasons: (1) CMV probably plays a major role in the underlying immune deficiency; and (2) life-threatening CMV infections occur in about 25% of people with AIDS.[6] Now that PWAs are living longer, the incidence of life-threatening CMV infections will probably increase.

DHPG and foscarnet are effective in controlling CMV. Unfortunately, both are toxic and, DHPG requires the implantation of a Hickman or similar catheter for intravenous administration.

Community-based research is exploring two exciting approaches to the prevention of CMV infections.

The first is high-dose acyclovir. Many people with AIDS are already taking high-dose acyclovir (20 or more pills a day), and anecdotal reports suggest that this regimen prevents CMV retinitis.[7] Another exciting prospect is the prophylactic use of a new oral form of DHPG.[8] FIAC and HPMPC are two other drugs currently in development for the treatment and prevention of CMV.[9] The prevention of CMV infections would contribute significantly toward increasing long-term survival.

Toxoplasmosis ("Toxo")

Although not all PWAs are at risk for toxoplasmosis, central nervous system toxoplasmosis was found at autopsy in 32 out of 780 AIDS patients at Memorial Sloan-Kettering Cancer Center.[10] Preventing toxo would be a major breakthrough.

Dr. Joseph Sonnabend of CRI-New York and Dr. Dennis Israelski from a community research group in Redwood City, California, have written a toxo prophylaxis protocol that compares different doses of pyrimethamine (Daraprim), with or without folinic acid (leucovorin). Dr. Donald Armstrong of Memorial Sloan-Kettering Cancer Center has agreed to be principal investigator of this study, and plans are under way to seek funding to conduct this as a multicenter trial with other community-based groups.

If funding can be found, this study can begin immediately and within a year and a half we could know whether these drugs prevent toxoplasmosis.

Mycobacterium Avium Intracellulare (MAI), Also Known as Tuberculosis

When most people think of tuberculosis, they think of Camille. But Camille died of *pulmonary* TB. MAI is another just-as-deadly form of tuberculosis. MAI is found in up to 50 percent of people with AIDS.[11] Preventing MAI is an urgent priority, because it is a very difficult disease to treat once it has spread throughout the body.

The County Community Consortium of San Francisco has written an MAI prophylaxis protocol using clofazimine. CRI-New York is one of the sites currently enrolling PWAs in an MAI prophylaxis trial of rifabutin.

Other drugs that ought to be investigated for the prevention of MAI include: amikacin, clofazimine, and new European antibiotics such as roxithromycin and azithromycin.[12]

Cryptococcal Meningitis, Candidiasis, and Other Fungal Infections

Many people with AIDS aren't waiting for the results of clinical trials and have begun taking fluconazole and Itraconazole to prevent life-threatening fungal infections. Either antifungal agent should also prevent histoplasmosis and coccidioidomycosis, in addition to candidiasis and cryptococcal meningitis.

Fluconazole is a fairly safe antifungal medication manufactured by Pfizer that was approved by the FDA in January 1990.

Because Janssen Pharmaceutical's Itraconazole is so much cheaper than fluconazole (and may be just as effective), it is a prime candidate for a prophylaxis trial. Antifungal prophylaxis trials are being planned by community-based research organizations.

Parasitic Infections Such as Cryptosporidiosis

Cryptosporidiosis (or "crypto," as it is known in PWA slang) is a comparatively rare complication of AIDS. But because it is debilitating and often deadly, finding a cure for crypto would be a major breakthrough. Preliminary evidence suggests that Diclazuril (a chicken-feed pesticide) kills the crypto parasite with little toxicity to the human host. Hyperimmunized crypto-specific cow's milk has also shown some efficacy. Trials of both therapies are under way.[13]

Kaposi's Sarcoma (KS) and
Autoimmune Thrombocytopenic Purpura (ATP)

No one knows for sure why PWAs get KS and ATP. Some researchers have proposed that tumor growth factors[14] may be responsible for KS and that other substances carried in the blood may be responsible for ATP. If so, removing them from the blood through a process known as plasmapheresis may ameliorate or even prevent KS and ATP.

Exciting preliminary data suggests that plasmapheresis, when used in conjunction with staph-A columns (a filter over which the blood passes that attracts immune complex and autoantibodies that then stick to the filter) can lead to the regression of KS lesions. Funding for a clinical trial of plasmapheresis and plasmapheresis with staph-A columns (brand name: Prosorba) is being sought.

Plasmapheresis with staff-A columns is already an approved treatment for autoimmune thrombocytopenic purpura, a common complication of AIDS that involves easy bruising.

Other potential therapies for KS are also being talked about with great excitement on the PWA grapevine.

Wasting Syndrome

Proper nutrition is the basis of life. Many gravely ill people with AIDS lose the desire or the ability to eat. Fortunately, it is possible to provide all the nutrients a person needs through intravenous feeding. Several physicians have extended the lives of people with AIDS who have wasting syndrome by administering total parenteral nutrition (TPN).

An appetite stimulant known as Megace, manufactured by Bristol Myers, is being prescribed for those who are able to eat but have lost their appetites. A community-based clinical trial of Megace is underway, and preliminary results look promising.

Anemia

Many people with AIDS develop severe anemia from AZT. (Anemia also results on occasion from AIDS itself.) Erythropoietin is a substance produced by the body that can correct anemia. A Treatment IND permitting the distribution of erythropoietin (EPO) has been granted by the FDA.

▨ The cutting edge of AIDS treatment research is the growing network of more than twenty-five community-based research groups in the United States whose top priority is the prevention of opportunistic infections. The CRI movement is doing an end run around federal incompetence and indifference. Through community-based research, we can save our *own* lives. Anyone who wants to survive AIDS would be well advised to make contact with the community-based research group in his or her area. Volunteer to save your own life and keep abreast of the latest developments in research.

NOTES

1. Gold, Jonathan, M.D., *AIDS Treatment Information Newsletter*, 3:4 (April 1989).

2. Harrington, Mark, "Organizing Community-Based Clinical Trials: Models for the AIDS Epidemic," handbook for a conference sponsored by CRI-New York and the County Community Consortium of San Francisco, in New York City (July 7–9, 1989): 64–68.

3. Dr. Michael Lange of St. Luke's/Roosevelt Hospital in Manhattan has discovered that allergic reactions are drastically reduced when he starts PWAs on lower doses of Bactrim and slowly builds up to the full dose of two double-strength tablets daily.

In the transcript from a Columbia University AIDS forum entitled "AIDS: Improving the Odds 1988" (see note 4 below), Dr. Lange described how he sensitizes people to Bactrim:

[I] start with 5 cc's of pediatric suspension, which is the equivalent of one regular tablet. Give that once a day for three to five days, and then build up to 10 cc's twice a day, which is the equivalent of a double-strength tablet twice a day. And after ten to fifteen days, I change to double-strength tablets.

4. See Dr. Michael Lange, quoted in Columbia Gay Health Advocacy Project, "AIDS: Improving the Odds 1988," New York City (1989): 15.

5. Harrington, ibid.

6. Harrington, ibid.

7. Dr. Craig Metroka presented the intriguing results from a study of high-dose acyclovir that was effective in preventing CMV in sixty patients with AIDS who were followed for two years. According to Dr. Metroka,

Sixty patients, all with fewer than 150 T4-cells/mm3, were studied from December 1987 to January 1989. Mean [T-helper] count at entry was 75. No patients receiving 800 mg. of acyclovir every 4 hours (4800 mg/day) developed evidence of disseminated CMV. Three of the 9 patients who refused high-dose acyclovir developed invasive CMV. Deaths of the 3 acyclovir-treated patients were unrelated to CMV.

For further information, see Dr. Craig Metroka, "Possible Usefulness of High-Dose Acyclovir as Prophylaxis for CMV," *Montreal Abstracts*, M.B.P. 126 (June 1989): 176.

8. The saga of oral DHPG is a prime example of the failure of the American system of drug testing. According to John James's *AIDS Treatment News*, 89 (October 20, 1989):

Oral ganciclovir has existed for years. . . . A study published over two years ago showed that the drug could be given orally and produce a high enough blood level to inhibit CMV [Jacobson, M.A., et al., "Human Pharmacokinetics and Tolerance of Oral Ganciclovir," *Antimicrobial Agents and Chemotherapy* (August 1987): 1251–1254].

A clinical trial of oral ganciclovir for the prevention of CMV ought to be a top priority of AIDS research.

9. James, ibid. See also *AIDS Treatment News*, 76 (March 24, 1989).

10. Gold, ibid.

11. Harrington, ibid.

12. Harrington, ibid.

13. A recent issue of John James's invaluable *Treatment News* contained an excellent overview of cryptosporidium and potential therapies.

14. It has been two years since federal AIDS researcher Dr. Robert Gallo announced that his lab had isolated a tumor growth factor that may play a role in the development of Kaposi's sarcoma. No further information about KS growth factor has been released by the federal government. It is cruel for government researchers to dangle such a tantalizing prospect and then refuse to deliver.

GOING FOR THE GOLD

Curing AIDS

▨▨▨ I believe that a cure for AIDS is within sight. Having finished this book, I intend to concentrate exclusively on saving my own life. I hope to explore the feasibility of the Community Research Initiative of New York testing a multimodal treatment regimen.

I have given up any hope that the federal research effort will ever help me save my life. The outrageously poor quality of science belatedly brought to bear on finding treatments sends the message loud and clear that the lives of those of us affected by AIDS are not deemed worthy of America's best efforts.[1] The country that put a man on the moon first has refused to apply a moon-launch mentality to the formidable task of curing the immune deficiency that we call AIDS.

Federal AIDS treatment research has concentrated almost exclusively on stopping HIV. The plain truth is that the all-eggs-in-one-anti-retro-viral-basket approach of federal researchers has produced little of value for people with AIDS. Five anti-retrovirals have been thrown at AIDS with no success.[2] And yet the government's obsessive focus on anti-retrovirals continues, at the expense of serious research into preventing opportunistic infections and correcting non-HIV-related immune defects.

If HIV—a retrovirus—is "the cause" of AIDS, then anti-retroviral drugs that prevent HIV replication should make people better. The fact that this doesn't seem to be the case suggests, at a minimum, that we need to broaden our approach to therapies. We need to begin to search for ways to correct other pathological mechanisms.

My own physician, Dr. Sonnabend, has devised a treatment regimen that we both hope will be tested at CRI-New York. The multimodal approach will do what virtually every AIDS researcher says needs to be done—test many drugs and interventions *in combination* in an attempt to correct the many immune defects that characterize AIDS.

The multimodal regimen is based on the multifactorial theory of AIDS first proposed by Dr. Sonnabend.[3] As discussed in an earlier chapter, the multifactoral model for the development of AIDS proposes that AIDS results from a cascade of events. If the multimodal treatment approach can correct any one of the immune system defects, it may be able to stop—or reverse—the vicious cycle of immunosuppression, much as removing several dominos from a line can stop the dominos that come after it from being knocked down.

The multifactorial explanation for AIDS in gay men proposes that the main causes of the profound immunodeficiency in AIDS are a combination of CMV infection, EBV reactivation, and the immunological consequences of these infections, together with immune responses to foreign tissues, i.e. foreign cells in blood and semen. Controlling CMV and EBV activity is the most important goal of the multimodal treatment protocol.

The second major goal is removing immune complexes, interferon, and T-cell autoantibodies. These goals may be achievable using a number of currently available nontoxic drugs and techniques. Each drug or therapeutic procedure is intended to correct a specific defect and much thought has been given to the schedule of events.[4]

The immune systems of someone with AIDS has a number of well-established defects, including polyclonal B-cell hyperactivation; sustained levels of interferon and tumor necrosis factor; circulating immune complexes; herpes virus reactions (in particular CMV and EBV). The goal of the multimodal model is to correct each of these defects, in the hope that doing so will break the positive feedback loop of immune suppression.

Even those who believe that HIV is playing a central role in AIDS admit that controlling intercurrent infections (such as CMV and EBV) and correcting other defects might have beneficial effects.[5]

The first step in the multimodal model is the aggressive diagnosis and treatment of all known active infections. It doesn't make sense to try to cure AIDS itself while the body is battling treatable infections.[6] After treatment for all treatable conditions, prophylaxis must be instituted.

The next goal is to control CMV and EBV. Several approaches will be tried, alone or in combination: high-dose acyclovir; CMV-specific gamma globulin injections; transfer factor; and possibly low-dose oral DHPG.

To control Epstein-Barr virus reactivation (which plays a role in the B-cell hyperactivation characteristic of AIDS), very low doses of a potent cancer chemotherapy drug will be given.[7]

Concurrently, immune complexes will be removed through a combination of regular plasmapheresis with and without staph-A columns.[8]

Low-dose naltrexone will also be prescribed to help lower interferon levels.[9]

During the course of the trial, attention will be paid to proper nutrition and to psychosocial support. The trial may also include holistic components designed to enhance self-healing, including massage and visualization.

Unfortunately, the multimodal treatment protocol will be labor-intensive and expensive. Exclusive of the extensive lab work, the cost of the multimodal model could run as high as $20,000 for six months per person, based on the retail value of each of the components. Even if the multimodal approach doesn't cure AIDS, we should be able to learn a great deal from the trial about immune defects and how they interact.

⊠ I keep myself alive by imagining the day when the cure for AIDS is announced. I sometimes feel that my goal is to stay alive long enough to witness the AIDS equivalent of the Nuremberg trials, where the scientists who've squandered so much money and so many lives pursuing dead ends in AIDS treatment research will be held accountable. Mostly, though, I sustain hope by concentrating on alternatives to the failed federal AIDS treatment research effort.

I have a very clear vision of myself free of AIDS. My immediate goal is to see the lesion on my right wrist that I hate so much (because it is a constantly visible reminder that I'm sick) gone by January 1, 1991.

Maybe it's HIV dementia, but I really believe it's possible that I'll live to see the end of AIDS. I intend to fight until all the suffering is over. I, for one, believe that the multimodal model and the community-based research movement are the best hopes we have.

NOTES

1. The list of atrocities boggles the mind. Infants whose immune systems are deficient who have been enrolled in the infamous placebo trial ACTG 45 involving intravenous gamma globulin have been exposed to the risk of septicemia and other infections that can result from the insertion of an IV needle. Because the study involves intravenous administration of drug as well as placebo, the babies often have to be strapped down so they won't pull the needles out. The image of sick babies being strapped down and exposed to the risk of getting an infection merely so that researchers can give them worthless saline is stomach-turning. Is it any wonder that the federal government is unable to fill such trials? Not surprisingly, as of late 1989, only 41 out of a projected 366 infants have been enrolled in this study.

Another horror story was a "delayed treatment trial" of foscarnet for the treatment of "non-immediately-sight-threatening" CMV retinitis. Huh? We are in the realm of Orwellian doublespeak. Isn't "non-immediately-sight-threatening CMV retinitis" a contradiction in terms? And what, exactly, is "delayed treatment"? Imagine a nurse walking into the room and saying "You need treatment now, but we're going to delay it; we'll be back when your retinitis has advance a few more micrometers; we're going to watch it advance until it travels the arbitrary distance outlined in the protocol. Treatment will be delayed until after the CMV has traveled a certain distance down your retina." Not surprisingly, this government-sponsored trial is also having serious problems enrolling patients.

Those in federal AIDS trials who didn't die from toxic effects of the drugs being tested often died of preventable opportunistic complications. Many have died of preventable diseases because studies were designed to use death and progression of disease to measure the efficacy of a drug. For example, early federal AIDS trials actually *forbade* the use of any form of PCP prophylaxis.

In October 1989, several months after FDA approval of aerosol pentamidine, a person with AIDS died of PCP in a federal ddI trial. He wasn't receiving PCP prophylaxis. Embarrassed, Dr. Anthony Fauci (head of federal AIDS research) finally issued a memorandum requiring that all people with AIDS in federal trials receive PCP prophylaxis.

In a particularly gruesome federal AIDS treatment trial, people with full-blown AIDS, most of whom undoubtedly already have high levels of interferon in their blood, are being pumped full of alpha interferon and AZT. (This trial was still ongoing as late as November 1989.) When the patients develop dangerously low levels of white blood cells as a consequence of these two toxic drugs, federal researchers then gleefully inject them with a colony stimulating factor (GM-CSF) to see if this drug corrects the interferon/AZT-induced neutropenia!

As horrifying as this track record of atrocities is, one might be willing to overlook them if the lives needlessly sacrificed had contributed toward finding treatments that work. But after nearly a decade, all the massive federal AIDS bureaucracy has delivered is AZT.

2. The five anti-retroviral therapies that have been tried without much success are HPA-23, Suramin, ansamycin, foscarnet, and AZT. In addition, Ampligen was touted as being anti-retroviral, and when the results of several early trials were analyzed, people receiving Ampligen did worse than people receiving placebo! As I write this, the drug of the month is yet another toxic antiretroviral ddI, which I fear is simply a different version of a bad idea. The first reports of ddI-related deaths from pancreatitis have already surfaced.

3. See Sonnabend, J. A., Witkin, S. S., et al., "A Multifactorial Model for the Development of AIDS in Homosexual Men." *Annals N.Y. Acad. Sciences,* 437 (1984): 177; and also Sonnabend, J. A., "AIDS: An Explanation for Its Occurrence in Homosexual Men," in *AIDS and Opportunistic Infections of Homosexual Men,* P. Ma and D. Armstrong, eds. Stoneham, MA: Butterworth Publishers, 1989.

4. Other nontoxic drugs and procedures may be added to the multimodal model if and as new information becomes available. For example, CRI-New York is currently conducting a small trial of lentinan, an antiviral and immune-modulating substance extracted from shiitake mushrooms.

In vivo studies have suggested that hypericin (an extract from St. John's Wort) is significantly more anti-retroviral than AZT and significantly less toxic. CRI-New York is conducting an informal monitoring project of the effects of hypericin on PWAs.

Another CRI-New York–sponsored informal monitoring project is collecting data on the effects of antabuse.

5. Even those who believe HIV is the main cause of AIDS are now beginning to grudgingly acknowledge that CMV plays a major role in the development of AIDS. For example, a study on 108 HIV-positive hemophiliacs (published in the *Lancet* on July 8, 1989) found that those with CMV infection were two and a half times more likely to develop AIDS. The study also found that those who had CMV infections deteriorated more quickly than those who did not.

6. For example, the role of untreated, or improperly treated, syphilis in the overall immune deficiency of AIDS is an intriguing question. Because the tests that detect syphilis in someone with AIDS are unreliable, it may make sense to empirically treat everyone with high-dose IV penicillin to make sure that any syphilis is eradicated.

7. Researchers have observed that one unintended side effect of this particular chemotherapeutic drug is a reduction in B-cell activity. To avoid toxicity, the doses will be significantly lower than those regularly given to treat cancer.

8. See Kiprov, D. D., Lipper, R., et al., "The Use of Plasmapheresis, Lymphocytopheresis, and Staph Protein A Immunoadsorption As an Immunomodulatory Therapy in Patients with AIDS and AIDS-related Conditions," *J. Clin. Apteresis,* 3 (1986): 133.

There are slight but important differences between regular and Prosorba plasmapheresis; the combination should be more effective than either alone at removing immune complexes and other unwanted substances such as interferon from the blood.

9. Dr. Bernard Bihari of New York is writing for publication the results of his study which found that low-dose naltrexone reduces levels of circulating interferon and dramatically reduces the number of opportunistic infections in people with AIDS. Larger community-based trials involving low-dose naltrexone are in the planning stages. For a brief summary of the original naltrexone study, see Bihari, Bernard, et al., "Low-Dose Naltrexone in the Treatment of AIDS: Long-Term Follow-up Results," Fifth International AIDS Conference, Book of Abstracts, M.C.P. 62 (1989): 552.

AFTERWORD

▨▨▨ I had wanted to write a breathless, optimistic, hopeful how-to—to offer a recipe guaranteed to insure long-term survival. But as with most other aspects of AIDS, there are simply no conclusive answers.

After talking to dozens of other long-term survivors; after interviewing many doctors and AIDS researchers; after reviewing the literature on psychoneuroimmunology and long-term survival for other diseases, I still don't know for sure why some of us have survived AIDS.

When I lay out all the pieces of the puzzle, I can see patterns, but certainly no single pattern. I feel like a kid who has dumped out the contents of a box containing pieces of a jigsaw puzzle. During the three years of my search for answers to the enigma of survival—my own and others'—I have certainly found more pieces than I started with. And I have even managed to fit some pieces together. But try though I might, I can't quite make out the whole picture. And I can't even be certain that all the pieces of the puzzle were in the box to begin with or that all the pieces in the box were part of the puzzle I was trying to solve.

I have tried to resist the temptation to exaggerate the good news or to censor the grim realities. The brutal fact is that most people diagnosed with AIDS do die, and nothing—not even the exciting news that survival probabilities are expected to double by 1993—can or should deny the magnitude of the suffering and death caused by AIDS. When examining AIDS survival probabilities, it's not a question of whether the glass is half-full or half-empty; the question, rather, is whether or not we can find it within ourselves, after all the grieving, to celebrate the fact that there exists a small (but growing) percentage of long-term survivors.

I certainly enjoyed the chatty intimacy of meeting others who had walked an unmarked path alone only to discover that all the while, a few feet away but unbeknownst, others were walking beside. There was something tangible and reassuring about sitting face-to-face with others similarly situated.

The people I interviewed invigorated me emotionally, but they certainly offered no prescription for surviving that I or anyone else could reliably follow.

It is amazing to me that as I write this final chapter—more than two years after many of these interviews were conducted—all but four of the survivors profiled in this book are still alive and thriving. Gary Mackler died just shy of the three-year anniversary of his diagnosis; Emilio died in the summer of 1989, having survived nearly six years after his first KS lesion appeared; Eddie died in March 1990—more than four years after his first bout with PCP; and Dan Turner died in June 1990, eight years after his diagnosis.

I have included their profiles to make the important point that their deaths in no way detract from the fact that they were survivors. All four defied the grim predictions and struggled nobly to prove the doomsday scenarists wrong. The lessons their lives teach us are important for those living with AIDS, and the fact that each ultimately succumbed to AIDS in no way diminishes what they have to teach us.

▨ Writing this book has forced me to acknowledge that I haven't been taking my own advice lately. I've been afraid to say no to increasing obligations and I've allowed my health to suffer. But that is going to change. I'm clearing my political plate. I have already resigned from most of the AIDS organizations that I helped found. Now that this book has been completed, I intend to focus more on my own physical and emotional health and to pursue the non-HIV-focused, multimodal approach to treating my illness outlined in the previous chapter.

▨ Do I think I'll die from AIDS? It depends on what day of the week you catch me. Sometimes, dropping into bed, bone-weary with exhaustion after a day of mixing it up in the political arena, I hear the clear message of my body that death is ticking quietly within me. Noticing a new lesion recently, I broke into a cold sweat, frozen momentarily in the image of my imminent death. Other days, I allow my strategy of momentum—of presenting a moving target to death—to lull me into a sense that I'll live a more or less normal life span.

When I'm in a really good mood, I harbor the humorous fantasy that

I'm slated to die in some bizarre way that will have nothing to do with AIDS. For instance, while on a speaking tour, I attended the Mr. Northwest Leather contest. During the fantasy segment, Contestant #4 lost control of a huge motorcycle, which roared off the stage directly toward me. The engine was still racing furiously when the motorcycle caught on a lighting tree and stopped about one foot from where I sat. My immediate thought was "I can see the headline now: 'PWA Long-Term Survivor Dies in Freak S/M Motorcycle Accident!'" Though I was terrified at the time, the irony of such an end did make me smile. At least I could have said that AIDS didn't get me.

Ultimately, I know that even if I were to die tomorrow, I could still take pride in the fact that I have become a long-term survivor of AIDS. With a lot of hard work and lots of luck, I have beaten amazing odds. No one can ever take that away from me.

▨ I am soul-weary of AIDS—of having it, of fighting it, and of hearing and thinking about it. But even in dark moments, when doubt and hopelessness threaten to overwhelm, I am aware of an almost palpable will to live. The hysterical *joie de vivre* of Julia Child cooking videos, my cookie-cutter collection, the imminent release of Bette Midler's next album, and the secure sensation of my lover coming to bed sometimes make me want to weep with joy. I should miss them so, if I died.

The uncritical repetition of the myth that everyone with AIDS dies denies the reality of—but perhaps more important, the *possibility* of—our survival. I have stubbornly clung to the belief that I would be among the lucky—that I was different—that I would survive. I have railed against, and cursed, and challenged hopelessness wherever I have encountered it.

In the end, I'm convinced that it's as rational to have hope as it is to give up. If 97 percent of people diagnosed with AIDS are dead after five years, then 3 percent are still alive. I, for one, intend to remain among that prophetic minority.